The Pilates Method of Physical
and Mental Conditioning

Novels by Philip Friedman:

TERMINATION ORDER

ACT OF LOVE, ACT OF WAR

RAGE

The Pilates Method
of Physical and Mental
Conditioning

PHILIP FRIEDMAN and GAIL EISEN

Doubleday & Company, Inc., Garden City, New York

1980

Photographs by Philip Friedman and Gail Eisen

Library of Congress Cataloging in Publication Data

Friedman, Philip, 1944–
  The Pilates method of physical and mental
  conditioning

   1. Exercise. 2. Mind and body. 3. Pilates,
Joseph Hubertus. I. Eisen, Gail, 1942– joint
author. II. Title.
RA781.F69   613.7′1

DESIGNED BY MARILYN SCHULMAN

ISBN: 0-385-14490-3
Library of Congress Catalog Card Number 78–22629
Copyright © 1980 by Philip Friedman and Gail Eisen

This book is dedicated to
Joseph and Clara Pilates
and to
Romana Kryzanowska

Contents

List of Exercises

To neglect one's body for any other advantage in life is the greatest of follies.

Arthur Schopenhauer

It is the mind itself which shapes the body.

Friedrich von Schiller

as quoted by Joseph Hubertus Pilates

The authors want to thank the staff at the Pilates Studio in New York for their attention and instruction over the years and particularly for their patience and assistance while we were working on this book.

Particular thanks to Laurie Scandurra for her help with the pictures, to John Winters, and especially to Romana Kryzanowska, who so enthusiastically embodies the spirit of Joseph Pilates and who adds to it her own personal flair, insight, and good humor. This book—indeed the survival of the original Pilates Method—would have been impossible without her.

The photographs in this book are of Gail Eisen, Laurie Scandurra, and Philip Friedman. They were taken by Philip Friedman and Gail Eisen, and the prints were made by Sandra Hochhausen.

The leotards and shorts are by Danskin, designed by Bonnie August, to whom we also extend our special thanks.

The Pilates Method of Physical
and Mental Conditioning

of the best and most famous) have unevenly developed bodies and—off the stage—move awkwardly.

Listen to William Bales, who has been a prominent dancer and choreographer, and a teacher and trainer of dancers for more than forty years:

"Seventy-five percent of the students who come to me with prior training know only how to do steps. They know nothing about the body or energy or breathing; they know only mechanics and virtuosity.

"With standard gymnasium-type exercises and most dance training, weak muscles tend to get weaker and strong ones stronger. Without special training, we tend to use two or three times as much energy as we need to do a given movement. In dance class, the emphasis is on movement, not the body. Too many dancers don't learn to use their bodies."

Bales has a solution to this problem: the Pilates Method.

As Dean of the Division of Dance at the State University of New York's unique "conservatory within a college" at Purchase, New York, Bales supervised the design of the first building in the United States to be built exclusively for dance education. He made sure that among the special rehearsal halls and studios and theaters there were two large rooms constructed solely for teaching and practicing the Pilates Method. The method is required preparation for all dance students; the course is called "Body Correctives," and it is taught by Romana Kryzanowska, doyenne of the Pilates Studio and prime disciple of Joseph Pilates, who devised and developed the Pilates Method.

Dance professionals, especially the true leaders in the art, must train their students to meet continuous extreme demands on their bodies. They have to choose the best possible method of conditioning. It is no accident that so many of them have adopted the Pilates Method.

In 1954, George Balanchine—then artistic director of the New York City Ballet—was concerned about a young dancer named Jacques D'Amboise, already one of the brightest stars in the City Ballet's glittering galaxy.

"You have bad posture," D'Amboise remembers Balanchine telling him. "And your muscles are too big."

Balanchine's solution? He hauled a reluctant D'Amboise off to see Joe Pilates. Full of youthful pride, D'Amboise resisted the discipline Pilates tried to impose, but in the end he succumbed, returning to Joe's studio years later and regularly ever since, a confirmed devotee.

"Until I went to Pilates," he says now, sitting with relaxed grace, one leg casually over the other, knee on knee, "I was so tight I couldn't cross my legs."

D'Amboise, who is still a principal dancer with the New York City Ballet, and who succeeded William Bales as Dean of Dance at Purchase, goes on: "The Pilates Method makes me feel exhilarated and absolutely wonderful. The exercises are excellent for strengthening and stretching the entire body, especially the lower abdomen and back. If all people did the Pilates Method there would be a good deal less back trouble."

BodyChange

Joe Pilates didn't believe in what he called "unnatural exercise"—forcing the body into strained postures or pushing it to repeat the same motions over and over again to the point of exhaustion. His goal was mental and physical harmony: the realization of each person's physical capabilities and the correction of imbalances and weaknesses.

Pilates' emphases on restoring the body to true balance, on ease and economy of movement, and on a channeled flow of energy was central to the appeal his method had for the greatest figures in the development of dance in America—both modern and classical. Besides George Balanchine, Pilates' followers included Jerome Robbins, Martha Graham, Hanya Holm, and Ted Shawn. Ruth St. Denis, who was known as "the first lady of American dance," said about the Pilates Method:

"Not only is the body rejuvenated, but the mental and spiritual refreshment is beyond calculation."

That's perhaps the most exciting thing about the Pilates Method. Each time you do the movements, you come away feeling stimulated and renewed.

Refreshment Beyond Calculation

Too many exercise programs leave you drained and tired. They are boring to do, and because of that they encourage sloppiness. With no pleasure in the doing and exhaustion to look forward to when you're done, it's easy to miss a day, and then two, and then to stop bothering entirely.

Not so with the Pilates Method.

No day is exactly like any other, of course, and sometimes you'll feel less like exercising than others, but once you have some experience with the Pilates Method, you'll come to look forward to the stimulation it can provide. And as time passes, you will find that without conscious effort you are walking and sitting straighter, moving more gracefully. Your muscles will become firmer and sleeker, better shaped, stronger without being large and bulky. You will be more supple.

And you will be calmer and more relaxed, with a new sense of control and inner harmony.

These effects are subtle at first, and it takes time for them to develop, but they are real. Some of them appear so gradually that at first you may not notice them, except indirectly.

People comment on how good you look; your clothes fit differently. You don't have those daytime energy dips. A familiar chair suddenly feels strange, because you are sitting straighter. One day you realize it's easier to reach for something you've dropped in an awkward corner under your desk; another day you catch a glimpse of yourself in a mirror or a shop window and are surprised at how straight you are standing, without seeming at all stiff.

How does the Pilates Method bring about these changes? Surprisingly simply, as you will see in the chapters that follow.

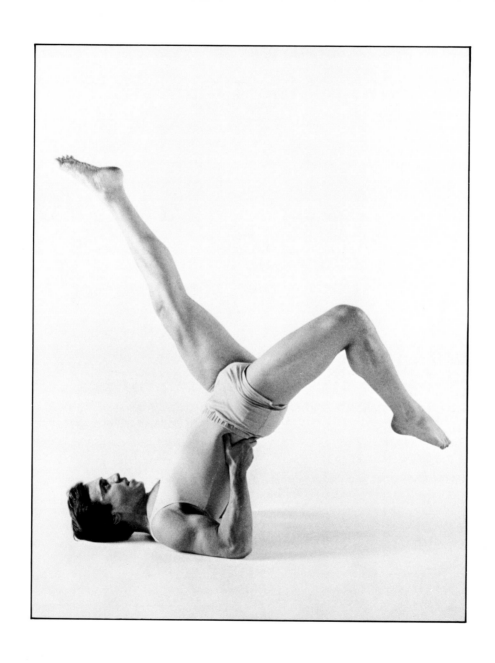

CHAPTER TWO

Something Different

Unlike most exercise programs, the Pilates Method follows carefully laid-out principles based on a well-constructed philosophical and theoretical foundation (one without mysticism or appeals to unseen forces, divine or otherwise). It is not merely a collection of exercises, it is truly a *method,* carefully developed and refined over a period of more than sixty years of use and observation.

For the Pilates Method to work properly for you, you have to be familiar with its basic principles from the beginning, before you start to do the movements.

Most important, the method relies on CONCENTRATION. To do the movements properly, you must pay attention to what you are doing. No part of your body is unimportant; no motion can be ignored.

The other watchwords (which will be explained in Chapter Three) are:

CONTROL
CENTERING
PRECISION
FLOWING MOVEMENT
BREATHING

Given the half-dozen basic principles embodied in these words, the Pilates Method can be summarized in a single sentence:

A few well-designed movements, properly performed *in a balanced sequence, are worth hours of doing sloppy calisthenics or forced contortions.*

It sounds simple, and in some important ways it *is* simple, but the changes it can work, not just in your body but in your life, are only a little bit short of miraculous.

East Does Not Meet West

Both physical and mental health have always been thought of as desirable, although standards and definitions of health and the relative importance of mind and body have varied with time and place.

In Western thought, in spite of occasional views of physical fitness as an aid to clear thinking (or—more commonly—of sickness and debilitation as an obstacle to thought), mind and body have been seen as separate. The Roman writer Juvenal embodied this perception when, two thousand years ago, he recommended praying for a sound mind in a sound body.

There have been some exceptions to this image, seeing a closer connection between mind and body, but it is only recently that physiologists have begun to investigate a possible mind-body linkage in a serious way, finding that exercise is accompanied by chemical changes in the blood and elsewhere in the body that may have important effects on brain function. Psychiatrists and psychologists are exploring connections between physical fitness and creativity, independence, self-esteem, and freedom from tension.

This is early scientific confirmation of ideas which have recently been grafted onto Western physical training from the East. Popular manuals for recreational sports are heralding the value of a new kind of cooperation between mind and body. For the first time, sports training is moving away from the old image of a highly motivated mind giving orders to a reluctant and sometimes recalcitrant body.

Even with these insights, the new approaches to mind-body linkages remain very Western, evoking touch football on the lawn, marathon races and tennis tournaments, and Polar Bear Club outings in the icy winter surf.

That is not the only way to look at the unity of mind and body. Consider Yoga and T'ai Chi, or the way archery and fencing can be embodiments of Zen Buddhism every bit as pure and spiritual as the tea ceremony or flower arranging. This kind of mysticism—seeing mind and body as aspects of the same entity, ideally in complete harmony—is common in the East, where physical training (rarely strenuous) can be one of many roads to an essential calmness and a sense of being centered and whole: at one with yourself and the world. The object of physical discipline is essentially religious and spiritual, rather than what Westerners would call "mental."

Of the Eastern disciplines, Yoga has the greatest following in this country, in various forms, some of them very modified. This following has by and large been separate from the segment of the population that enjoys recreational and competitive sports. Yoga and its relatives are basically static: they emphasize rest, contemplation, stretching, and limberness, while Western physical activities—from basketball to ballet—are dynamic and kinetic, emphasizing motion, muscle tone, and strength.

All of these activities have their benefits, if they are pursued regularly and faithfully, but they have their drawbacks as well. Traditional Western methods of physical training strengthen without true control, and they emphasize physical imbalances. Strong muscles get stronger while weak ones, unconsciously avoided, get weaker. Eastern methods are better at producing relaxation and suppleness, and if you follow them far enough they can give you extraordinary control of certain muscles, but they do little for muscle tone or endurance. Yoga, in particular, stretches without strengthening most parts of the body; its more advanced postures may lead to pain and injury by twisting joints and tendons beyond their normal limits. Also, movement and contemplation tend to be separate in the Eastern systems; as a result, tranquillity and "wholeness" come to be associated with stopping and taking a break from other activities.

Each of these approaches—Western and Eastern—fails to produce the benefits of the other. It is hard to combine them, because in many ways they are incompatible. And the answer isn't to do them both, because they're not really complementary; you're more likely to end up with the drawbacks of both approaches than all of their benefits.

What is needed is something different, a system that starts with more unified assumptions and goals.

The Best Method

In the eighteenth century, the great German poet and philosopher Friedrich von Schiller said, "It is the mind (*Geist*) itself which builds the body."

Joseph Pilates was fond of quoting that line. More than sixty years ago, it led him to begin developing a system of conditioning based on the principle that the body must be actively trained and controlled through the discipline of the mind. His aim was to make people more aware of themselves, more in touch with their whole, integrated being—to bring body and mind together into a single, dynamic, well-functioning entity.

In a sense, he was trying to capture the best effects of both the Western and Eastern approaches to physical and mental conditioning in a unified, consistent system. It is a measure of his genius that he succeeded.

BodyChange

The Pilates Method changes bodies. It makes them fitter and stronger and more attractive. It slims the muscles and makes them more compact, developing sleekness rather than bulk. It turns the abdomen and lower back and hips into a firm central support for a newly supple and graceful body. It sets up no artificial standards of performance. And its effects are more than just physical.

Not long ago, Romana Kryzanowska was teaching a movement to a woman who was at the Pilates Studio for her third session. "You know, Romana," the woman said, "I do Transcendental Meditation. And that's what this is. It's Transcendental Meditation."

Of course, it isn't TM. But the woman's comment is an important one. Because while the Pilates Method is effectively toning muscles, it is also working to produce a remarkable unity of body and mind, a wholeness comparable to that claimed by TM and other meditation systems. But the Pilates Method operates without mysticism or exaggerated self-consciousness. Unlike the Westernized versions of Eastern disciplines, the Pilates Method recognizes that these mental changes are blocked if too much attention is paid to them. They have to grow naturally. They cannot be forced.

In the Pilates Method, the emphasis is on *doing* and *being*. Your mind is directed toward your body, concentrating on what is happening as it happens. Learning, growth, and integration, like the changes in the shape of your body, are brought about by the activity itself, without conscious stress on the goals.

You worry about the present; the future takes care of itself.

Light and Fluid and Energizing

Everything about the Pilates Method is flowing and buoyant.

In each motion, you go only as far as you can, up to the point where you first feel strain, and then you go on to something else. The movements are done a few times each (usually three to five, rarely more); there is no boring repetitiveness. You learn to feel, to know exactly what your body is doing.

Exercise is more pleasant when your mind is totally engaged with your body. Concentrating over a period of time on centering, control, precision, flowing motion, and breathing results in the growth of a powerful sense of well-being and confidence.

Other systems of exercise quickly become boring, mostly because you have no sense of involvement in what you are doing. All you care about is getting through a certain number of repeated motions in a certain time. It doesn't matter how you do the motions, as long as you finish. Distractions—music, counting aloud—are the only relief.

That kind of exercise is inefficient, and it is almost impossible to enjoy. The best that most people can do with it is to achieve a sweatily masochistic pleasure from the spectacle of their own straining.

The Pilates Method is different. It merges your mental and physical processes so that you aren't an observer, watching yourself do difficult motions, but rather you are a participant.

When you finish a Pilates workout, you feel refreshed and invigorated. Energized. Every muscle has been stretched and toned and massaged.

Pilates Leads the Way

Joe Pilates used to say, "When I'm dead, they'll say, 'He was right.' I'm fifty years ahead of my time."

He was doubly right—in his method, and in his prediction.

He brought the basic concepts to this country when he arrived from Germany with Clara, a nursery and kindergarten teacher he met on the boat on the way to America and later married. They had been drawn together by a mutual interest: "We talked so much about health and the need to keep the body healthy," Clara said years later. "We decided to open a physical fitness studio."

It was far from Joe's first experience as a teacher. He had already taught self-defense to detectives in England, and then, with the outbreak of World War I, self-defense, wrestling, body-building, and rehabilitation to fellow internees in Lancaster and on the Isle of Man. After the war, he returned to Germany and was training the Hamburg police when an invitation to train the new German Army convinced him it was time to leave for America.

Joseph Hubertus Pilates was born in 1880 near Düsseldorf. Like many others who went on to excel physically, he was a frail child. Worries about tuberculosis led him to work so hard at body-building that by fourteen he was posing for anatomy charts. And studying them avidly.

A diver, skier, and gymnast in Germany as a teen-ager, Joe decided in 1912 to go to England, where he was a boxer and circus performer as well as an instructor in self-defense. When, at the outbreak of war, he was interned with other German nationals in England, he used what was for others a period of forced idleness to develop and refine his ideas about health and body-building. He boasted later that because they followed his regimen not a single one of his fellow internees had been laid low by the influenza epidemic that killed thousands in England in 1918.

It was in Germany in the early twenties that his work first took hold in the world of dance, when he met Rudolph von Laban, originator of Labanotation, the most widely used form of dance notation. Laban incorporated some of Joe's body-building techniques into his own teaching. It was from him

that Hanya Holm first learned of Joe's work, which she made part of the regular warm-up in the Holm technique.

And so the Pilates Method began to spread and to be diluted. Some of his early disciples merged his work into their own. Inevitably, pieces of the method were carried away by their students, who, without the underpinnings of direct contact with the master, shifted the emphasis and distorted the movements so that Joe himself would barely recognize them. Even his name was borrowed: there are dance-class warm-ups which are widely called the "Pilates," the way table tennis is called Ping-Pong. Many of the most glamorous and successful entrepreneurs of exercise have drawn heavily from Joe's work. Both the Nickolaus Method and Ron Fletcher's Beverly Hills emporium of "Body Contrology," acknowledge their debt to Pilates. ("Contrology" is a word originally coined by Pilates to describe his own theories and method.)

Ted Shawn, one of the founders of the famous dance center at Jacob's Pillow, Massachusetts, said about Joe: "Pilates has never received the recognition commensurate with his greatness."

Of course, that judgment depends on how you measure recognition. Joe Pilates had an important influence on most of the major innovators in dance in America, and his followers have included (and still include) a staggering roster of people prominent not only in dance, but in the theater and movies, in music, in business, medicine, and society; people whose bodies (and minds) are their professional stock in trade, and people for whom beauty and vitality are a way of life.

A full list of Pilates Studio regulars is impossible; a few examples past and present, give an idea of the spectrum: Suzanne Farrell, Maria Tallchief, Tanaquil LeClercq; Jacques D'Amboise, Ivan Nagy; Bambi Linn and Rod Alexander; Lauren Bacall, Katharine Hepburn, Jill Clayburgh, Candice Bergen, Laurence Olivier, Eddie Albert, José Ferrer, Tony Roberts; Gian-Carlo Menotti, Yehudi Menuhin, Roberta Peters; Francesco Scavullo; François de la Renta, Mica Ertegun, Jean Murray Vanderbilt; some people named Gimbel and Guggenheim; a smattering of counts and countesses.

Some of them have been coming regularly to the Pilates Studio for more than twenty years. Others, out-of-towners, come whenever they are in New York and talk enthusiastically about how glad they are to be back.

The Secret Revealed

Joe Pilates was jealous of the system he spent so much time and effort developing. He was willing enough to teach it himself, but he was reluctant to entrust it to others. Romana Kryzanowska and John Winters, now the senior instructors at Pilates Studio, worked with Joe and Clara for decades, but he remained the sole master of Pilates Studio, working with undiminished energy well into his eighties.

Until now, no serious effort has been made to embody the Pilates Method in a book that can be used in the home by people who have never been to the studio. It was clear that the project could not be undertaken except by long-time students of the method, and that the book itself would have to be different in some ways from the familiar format of books that offer instruction in physical fitness.

What's in This Book?

Having introduced you to Joe Pilates and his method, we're going to move on to a more complete description of the six basic principles that are the core of the Pilates Method. Then we will give you some experiments you can do with your body, to help you learn more about how it moves and what it does when you're not paying close attention to it.

In a way, the next two chapters (Three and Four) are the most important part of the book. If you master them, you can apply the knowledge you've gained in areas of your life beyond the method itself. (We'll say more about that later.)

Chapter Five is for getting ready. In it you'll learn how to approach the exercises themselves, and what preparation and equipment are necessary. And we'll point out a few basic cautions.

Next is the method itself, presented in two chapters. Chapter Six gives ten of the Pilates Method movements: a routine that will train you in the method and at the same time begin to produce beneficial results. Chapter Seven is the full program of mat exercises, coded so that you can build at your own pace from the basic routine of ten exercises until you are doing the entire sequence.

As the method grew, Joe invented apparatus to supplement it, and movements were added that are not part of the basic sequence. Some of these can be adapted so that you can do them without the apparatus. We've put them in Chapter Eight. Chapter Nine takes you away from the mat, introducing movements you can do to refresh yourself at the office or on a trip or wherever you are. In Chapter Ten you'll find a few words about the Pilates Method and some popular sports, both outdoor and indoor.

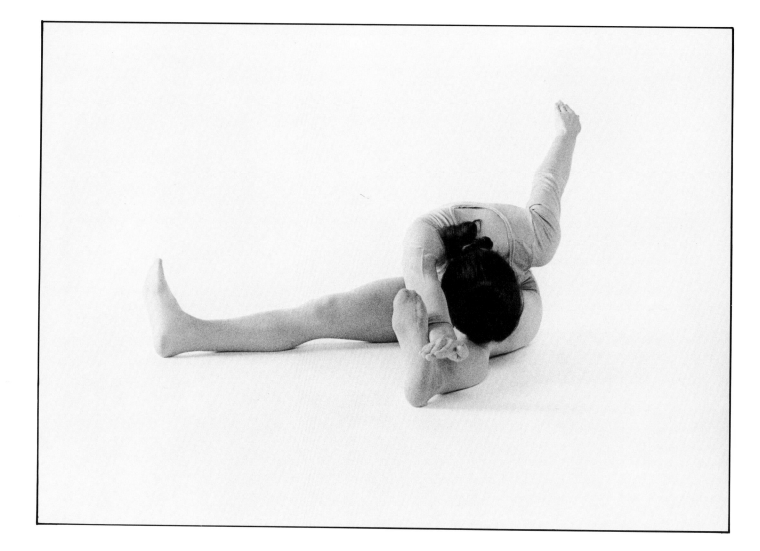

CHAPTER THREE

Mind Over Matter

The most important thing is not what you do but how you do it.

This may seem an odd thing to say about a system of movements as carefully designed and coordinated as the Pilates Method, but we are not talking here about the triumph of style over substance.

The central element of the Pilates Method is also its most paradoxical. The method's goal (beyond slimming and strengthening) is to create a fusion of mind and body, so that *without thinking about it* you will move with economy, grace, and balance; you will hold yourself regally; and you will use your body to the greatest advantage, making the most of its strengths, counteracting its weaknesses, and correcting its imbalances. The paradox is this: to produce an attention-free union of mind and body, the method requires that you constantly pay attention to your body while you are doing the movements. This attention-paying is so vital that it is more important than any other single aspect of the movements or the method.

The way you pay attention as you do the Pilates exercises takes a specific form. There are six basic principles of the Pilates Method; they were named in Chapter Two. Here, they'll be explained a little more fully.

CONCENTRATION

"Study carefully and do slowly the foundation work," Joe wrote once, in his characteristic Pilatean diction. "Follow directions exactly, with respect to every detail given."

You have to concentrate on what you're doing. All the time. And you must concentrate on your entire body.

This is not something you'll be able to do when you start, because it's harder than you think. Once you begin really to pay attention to your body, you will find that a movement which may have seemed simple is actually quite complex.

Here's an experiment you can do right now:

Put your right hand out at your side, straight out from the shoulder, with your fingers pointed. Bend your elbow and touch the tip of your forefinger to your nose.

Now, do it again, concentrating on what is happening to your arm. Does your elbow drop or rise as you move your hand? Do you turn your wrist? At what point? When you're touching your nose with your forefinger, what is the position of your other fingers?

What about your head? Was it straight or tilted? Chin up, down, or level? Did you turn it as you moved your hand and arm? What were you looking at?

Now do it with both arms at once. Ask yourself the same questions. Do it again, paying enough attention to be able to answer all the questions as you do the movement.

That's a lot to think about, and we haven't even begun to talk about the position of your chest and back and stomach and legs and how they're affected by what you've been doing.

The first thing you'll learn, doing the Pilates Method, is that the position and movement of every part of your body is interrelated and important. When you're walking, how you place your foot both influences and is affected by the way you hold your head.

Concentrating on your whole body at once as it performs complicated movements is a formidable challenge, but it is a skill that will come to you, a step at a time, as you pursue the Pilates Method. And once you have it, you will find that it's a remarkably valuable resource: an aid to both work and relaxation, and the key to an effortless fusion of mind and body.

CONTROL

Nothing about the Pilates Method is haphazard. The reason you need to concentrate so thoroughly is so you can be in control of every aspect of every movement. Not just the large motions of your limbs, but the positions of your fingers and head and toes, the degree of arch or flatness of your back, the rotation of your wrists, the turning in or out of your legs.

Most of our early experiences in school gyms have allowed us—in some cases, encouraged us—to fling ourselves around more or less indiscriminately. Think about doing a "jumping jack," for instance, or the legs-spread toe-touching exercise sometimes called a "windmill." What was there of grace or control in those, or in any other of the calisthenics you did?

This sloppiness carries over into our everyday life, and especially into recreational sports. It would be a lot easier for a golfer to keep his head down through his swing if he were not accustomed to letting it simply flop around every time he made a sweeping and largely uncontrolled motion of his arms and shoulders. And motion without control can lead to injury.

Our second watchword will be "control."

Suzanne Farrell is principal dancer with the New York City Ballet and a guest soloist of worldwide renown. She is someone whose control of her body is as complete as anyone could want. Her ballet training and her talent give her the consummate skill that has made her reputation. But, like Jacques D'Amboise and others we have mentioned, she builds on a more fundamental foundation. She explains: "The Pilates Method teaches you to be in control of your body and not at its mercy."

riage. A properly developed center can also mean less fatigue and a lowered incidence of back pain and injury. (It is widely recognized that suppleness and balanced strength in the lower back are important preventives of the chronic lower back pain that has become a major health problem in this country.)

In the instructions for the Pilates movements, we refer repeatedly to establishing a firm center and to techniques which are intended to help you develop and strengthen your center. Sometimes, when people see something over and over again, they get the impulse to say, "Oh yeah, that again," and then slide by to the next thing. In this case, don't do that. If you do, you'll be missing a lot.

CENTERING

Our first requirement in concentrating on our bodies and gaining full control of them is a starting place: somewhere to begin building our own bodily foundation.

Consider the part of your body that forms a continuous band, front and back, between the bottom of your rib cage and the line across your hipbones. We call this your "center." (This is not the same as the "center" of Yoga or other Eastern disciplines. It is a physical, not a mystical center.)

The center is the focal point of the Pilates Method. Firming and strengthening your center while keeping it stretched and supple is the prime physical result of practicing the method, and what a glorious result it is! It means a trimmer waist and flatter belly; it means better posture and a more regal car-

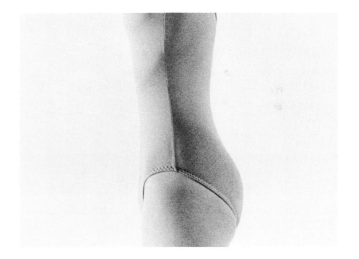

FLOWING MOVEMENT

In describing the essence of a Pilates movement, Romana Kryzanowska frequently speaks of "flowing motion outward from a strong center."

Nothing should be stiff or jerky. Nothing should be too rapid or too slow. Smoothness and evenly flowing movement go hand in hand with control.

PRECISION

Precision is another vital partner of control.

"Concentrate on right movements each time you exercise," Joe Pilates said, "else you will do them improperly and lose their value."

Haphazard movement can be useful for certain kinds of muscle building: there is nothing precise in the popular image of "pumping iron." But concentrating on precision of motion and precision of placement creates a kind of bodily fine tuning that carries over into everyday life as grace and economy of movement.

BREATHING

Breathing is the last on our list so that it will be one of the first in your mind.

Pilates believed in getting the blood pumping so that it could awaken all the cells in your body and carry away the wastes that are related to fatigue. For the blood to do its work properly, it has to be charged with oxygen and purged of waste gases, and that means proper breathing.

Full and thorough inhalation and exhalation are part of every Pilates exercise. Joe saw forced exhalation as the key to full inhalation. "Squeeze out the lungs as you would ring a wet towel dry," he used to say. "Soon the entire body is charged with fresh oxygen from toes to fingertips, just as the head of steam in a boiler rushes to every radiator in the house."

Here, too, we're concerned with concentration and control and precision. Breathing should be properly coordinated with movement.

Each exercise is accompanied by breathing instructions. In addition, there are a few general principles that will help when you're doing something that doesn't come with breathing instructions attached.

"Breathe in on the point of effort," Romana Kryzanowska advises, "and out on the return or relaxation." This is a rule that is sometimes modified by the form of the activity: If you're doing something that squeezes your body tight, use the motion to squeeze air out of your lungs and inhale when you straighten up.

And always remember the words of Uncle Joe: "Even if you follow no other instructions, learn to breathe correctly."

The Ruling Principles at Work

We can make all this clearer by looking at a simple motion, one you're almost certainly familiar with. It's a standard gym-class exercise, and it appears in some form in virtually every book on exercise or physical culture. It's usually called a "leg lift." It's not, by itself, a Pilates movement, but we've adapted instructions from movements of which it's a part so you can demonstrate to yourself the principles that have been discussed in this chapter.

You should do the following experiment lying on a soft or well-padded rug, or on an exercise mat. (See Chapter Five.)

First, try a leg lift the ordinary way:

1. Lie flat on your back with your hands at your sides.
2. Raise one leg until it is perpendicular to the floor (at a ninety-degree angle) or as close as you can get.
3. Lower it to the floor again.

Not a very hard motion, although most people find it a problem to get their leg even close to a ninety-degree angle with the floor.

Chances are, though, that when you were doing it, you:

1. arched your back
2. arched your neck
3. bent the knee of the leg you were raising
4. bent the other knee

5. rolled a little to one side or the other, or both
6. stuck your stomach out
7. held your breath
8. lifted your hips from the mat

All of these things make a difference: They reduce the effectiveness of the motion. They can, potentially, cause problems.

If you do ten or twenty such leg lifts, as is frequently suggested by gym teachers, coaches, and exercise books, you'll surely be tired and sweaty, but you will not have done yourself much good—certainly not in proportion to the effort you will have expended—and you might well end up cramped and stiff. Worse still, if you're prone to back pain or similar problems, that kind of jerky and uncontrolled motion is liable to aggravate it.

Now, let's look at (and try) the same motion, the way it would be done following the basic Pilates principles.

In the Pilates Method, any movement like this will begin by establishing a *strong center,* firmly anchored, and moving outward from this center.

A strong center is the focus of all the Pilates movements. It appears in different forms, but it is always there. It is the foundation on which your new fitness, grace and suppleness will be built.

1. Lie flat on your back, with your hands at your sides, palms on the floor.

2. Press your spine flat against the mat.

3. Try to make your navel touch your spine. (Visualize a very heavy weight on your stomach, pressing your entire midsection down toward the mat.) Do not suck in your stomach by holding your breath. Keep breathing normally.

The entire middle part of your body, from your hips to your shoulders, should feel *anchored* to the mat. The most important thing is to retain this feeling of *firmness* and *anchoring* throughout the movement.

At this point, if you have followed the first three instructions, your knees are probably slightly bent, your shoulders and arms may be tense, and your neck is likely to be arched. These side effects are natural, but they are not what we want, so we'll take care of them next.

Continuing to maintain your firmly anchored, strong center, and continuing to breathe evenly and normally:

1. Relax your shoulders and arms.

2. Your head is resting on the mat. Rotate it forward so that its point of contact with the mat is as close to your neck as possible (your chin will move toward your chest). Think of making your neck long and straight. Press the base of your skull into the mat.

3. Stretch your heels as far away from your hips as you can. (feel your knees straighten?) Keeping your heels stretched out, bend your feet back; try to point your toes at your head. (We call this "flexing" your feet.)

Is your spine still flat on the mat? Remember—press down spine and stomach.

Next:

1. Relax your right foot. Stretch the toe as far away from your hip as it will go. Don't cramp your foot over like a ballet dancer. Just let the toe lead your leg away from your hip.

2. Keeping your spine anchored to the mat and your toe stretched out, raise your foot as high off the mat as it will go. *At the same time, breathe in deeply and evenly.*

3. Pause with your foot raised. Flex your raised foot. (Push the heel away from your hip and pull the toe back toward your head.)

4. Keeping your heel pushed out, lower your leg slowly toward the mat. *At the same time, breathe out forcefully and evenly.* Press all the air from your lungs.

NOTE: As you raise and lower your foot, remember the heavy weight pressing down on your middle. Don't let your stomach bulge out.

Clearly, this is very different from the ordinary leg lift we started with. It's not hard to see how much more it does for you, and it's obvious, too, that learning to do one of these Pilates-style leg lifts, with the proper concentration and control, paying attention to your centering, flowing motion, precision, and breathing, will provide benefits you could never get from doing any number of sloppy gym-class leg lifts.

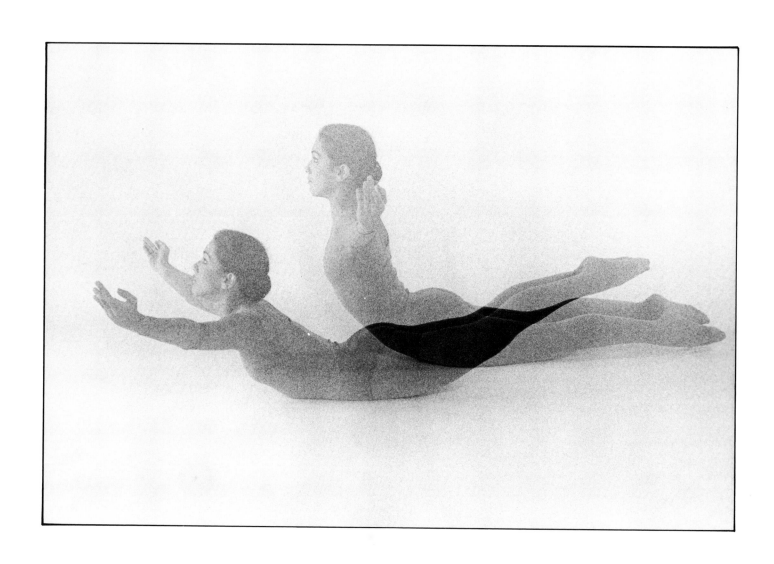

CHAPTER FOUR

Finding Your Body

"Okay, folks. Time to do our setting-up exercises for today. First off, we're going to touch our toes. Okay, let's go—up and down and up and down. Let's get some stretch into it."

Obviously, if you've read this far, you know that's not the way to begin.

The right way, the way that will do some good, is to start by getting in touch with how your body moves and to learn something about the ways you can control it.

We call this "finding your body," and it's an absolutely vital first step.

Finding your body will make it possible for you to get the most out of the Pilates Method movements described in the chapters to come, and it will also—even at this early stage—begin to change the way you think about your body and the way you move all day long.

In this chapter, we will also introduce some key words and phrases that will appear regularly in what follows, and we'll explain the special meanings they have for moving the Pilates way.

Where's Your Body?

Most of the time, we have little or no sense of what our body is doing. We may know that we're sitting or standing, legs crossed or not, but what about the position of our head and neck? Our shoulders?

Take a moment and try to visualize all the parts of your body without looking up from the page. Get a mental picture of the position of your feet and legs, your hips and buttocks, your stomach (by which we mean the part of your abdomen in the vicinity of your navel). Visualize your spine and back. Your shoulders. Your chest. Your neck and head.

Pay particular attention to your stomach, spine, neck, head, and shoulders. Where is your stomach in relation to the frame of bone that forms your hips? Lean forward slightly. Feel your hips tilt and your stomach shift position. Does your neck continue the line of your spine, or does it jut forward? What about your shoulders? Are they level or tilted? Shrug them up as high as you can and then let them drop of their own weight. Are they lower than they were? Let them drop still farther. Don't force them down, just think of loosening the muscles that you used to shrug them.

If you are sitting, push yourself all the way back in the chair so that the base of your spine touches the back of the chair. Flatten your back against the chair a little at a time, starting at the base of your spine and working your way smoothly upward. Where are your shoulders? Let them drop lower if they've risen.

It's likely that this position feels stiff and uncomfortable to you now. After some experience with the Pilates Method, it will seem much more natural.

RELAXING

It's important to establish a difference in your mind between relaxing and simply collapsing or falling apart.

There is a tendency some people have when learning the Pilates Method: because of the emphasis on control and precision, they tense up too much, using far more effort than is actually necessary; in essence, they are overcontrolling. If you are at the Pilates Studio and you do this, an instructor can point it out to you. Doing the method at home, alone, you will have to watch for it yourself, unless you have a partner.

The cure for this overtension is to relax the muscles while maintaining enough tone to hold the position you want.

Try this: lift your right arm and hold it in front of you with your elbow loosely bent and your fingers drooping toward the floor. Now straighten your fingers and reach outward with your fingertips so your arm straightens. (Hold your shoulder in place.) Keep reaching with the very tips of your fingers until your arm can stretch no longer and then tense all the muscles in your arm. Your arm should feel rigid. It may even be shaking.

Now, without changing the position of your fingertips, reverse the process you have just gone through. Untense the muscles of your arm, still holding it straight. You will reach a point where your elbow unlocks but your arm is still straight. If you relax further, you reach the point of collapse: your arm will drop or your elbow will bend.

When we talk about relaxing in this book, we mean removing the tension in your muscles while retaining tone and control. We do not mean collapsing.

EXPLORING THE CENTER

The center, as we've said, is that vital area between the bottom of your rib cage and the line across your hips. Joe Pilates called it the body's "powerhouse." For most of us, it is the most neglected part of our bodies, and it is the site of our two most vexing fitness problems. One problem is in front of us, and we're very aware of it—that perennially unflat belly. The other is behind us, and we're less aware of it until it becomes a source of pain and sometimes immobility—a too-frequently weak, stiff, and an unevenly developed lower back.

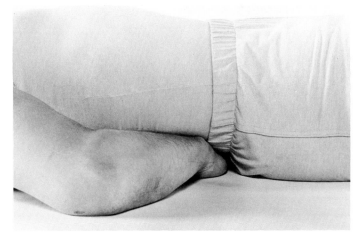

Lie down on a soft rug or exercise mat with your legs straight, your feet together, and your arms at your sides. Naturally, there will be a large space under the small of your back.

Put your hand between your back and the mat. It really goes in there, doesn't it? Press your back down against your hand. Feel the muscles at work.

Take your hand out. Press your back down against the mat. Are you still using the same muscles? Relax so that your back returns gradually to its earlier position. Be aware of the muscles you are using.

NAVEL TO SPINE

This is a phrase you'll be seeing a lot in this book. It is Pilates Method shorthand for making the distance between your stomach and back as small as possible. It's important not to confuse this with the kind of "sucking in your gut" beloved of gym teachers and drill instructors. Above all, you must never hold your breath.

Start out lying down. Visualize a large weight on your stomach. Let it press your stomach flat. Keep breathing normally. Now visualize a mattress button in your navel, with a string running through your body to your spine. Tighten the string, pulling your navel toward your spine. Keep breathing without letting your stomach rise at all. Your ribs will rise and fall to make room for the air in your lungs, but hold your stomach flat. Think of actually making your navel touch your spine. Feel the tension in your abdominal muscles. Keep breathing normally. Relax gradually.

Sit up with your knees bent comfortably. Let your head drop forward. Think of the mattress button in your navel again and watch your stomach as you tighten the string, drawing your navel closer to your spine. Again, keep breathing without letting your stomach bulge out. Make yourself as thin as you can and then gradually relax your abdominal muscles.

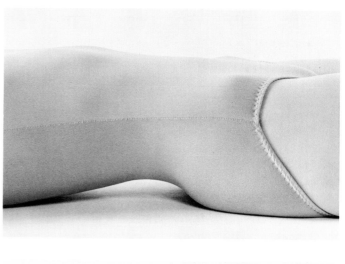

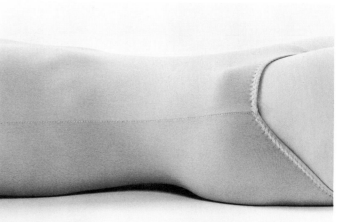

SPINE TO MAT

"Spine to mat" is another very important phrase, frequently combined with "navel to spine."

Lie down again. Legs straight, feet together. As you did before ("Exploring the Center"), press your back as flat as you can. Try to get all the air out from under it. Check by seeing if you can get your fingers under the small of your back. If you can, leave them there, and try to squash them between your back and the mat. Feel the muscles work. Take your hand away without relaxing the muscles which are pressing your back toward the mat. Press harder.

Now, still without relaxing your back, bend your knees and move your feet in toward your body. Your back will automatically press more strongly into the mat. Feel it flatten. Try to get your hand under your back now. Does it go as far?

Bend your knees still more and press your navel toward your spine. Feel yourself anchored to the mat all along your back. Now, if you can, raise your feet high off the mat and straighten your legs. They should be pointing more or less at the ceiling. Your back should still be flat against the mat. Check with your hand. (Remember to keep your navel pressed toward your spine and to keep breathing normally.)

Lower your legs a little toward the floor, keeping your back anchored. Is your back still flat?

Testing with your hand, lower your legs until the small of

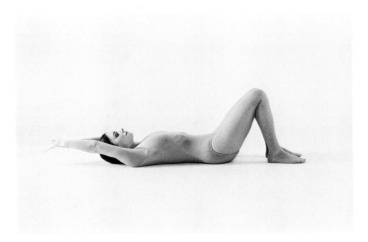
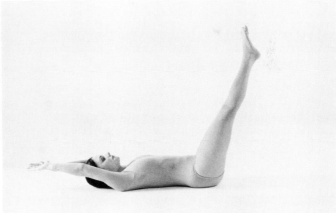

your back lifts off the mat. As soon as it does, lower your legs immediately to the mat. Relax, but don't collapse!

For everyone, there is a point at which lowering the legs makes the back arch up off the mat this way. The stronger your center, the lower you can get your legs before this happens.

It's a good idea to do this experiment several times (not necessarily all at once; don't strain), making small adjustments upward and downward in the position of your legs, until you have a good sense of how far you can go and still comfortably maintain your anchored position on the mat. At the beginning, it's likely that you will have to keep your legs quite high off the mat. Don't worry about it; improvement will come.

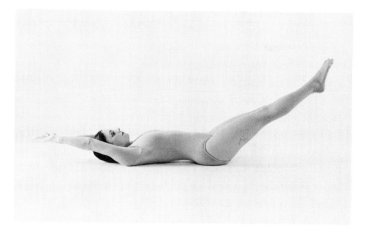

STRETCHING YOUR NECK

Lie on your back with your legs straight and your feet together. Press your spine to the mat and your navel to your spine. Keep breathing normally.

What is the position of your head and neck? Chances are your head is back and your neck is arched. Rotate your head forward and stretch your neck, trying to flatten the back of your neck to the mat. You can't, of course. All you can do is move the point of contact between your head and the mat from somewhere near the top of your skull to somewhere much nearer its base. This will automatically bring your chin in toward your throat.

There is a tendency, in adjusting the position of your head and neck, to tense your shoulders. You should be loose through your chest and shoulders.

This position of head and neck produces a sensation of lengthening or stretching your neck. For that reason, we will sometimes signal it by suggesting that you "make your neck long." Another key phrase is "press the base of your skull into the mat."

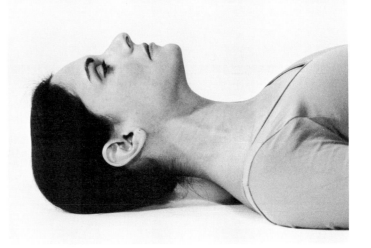

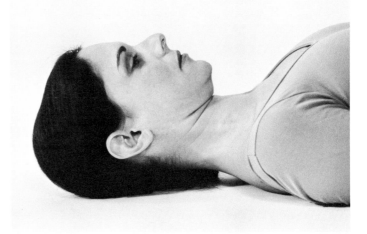

FOOT POSITIONS

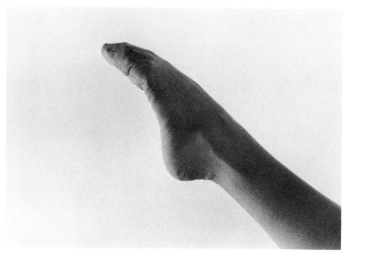

Like the head, the foot is a part of the body that's frequently left to flop around on its own, more or less neglected in both verbal and written exercise instructions. Sometimes a conscientious writer or instructor will specify "point your toes," but that's usually about it.

That's too bad, because, as you will see, the position of your feet can be very important indeed in how a movement feels and the benefit you get from it.

First, something to avoid: don't point your toes. That is, don't do what almost everyone does on receiving the instruction "point your toes," which is to curl their feet over into a tight position apparently meant to resemble a ballerina's toe shoe when she's on point. This throws your foot out of line in a way that interferes with your using your legs properly in the Pilates Method, and it can give you cramps in the muscles of your feet.

When we talk about pointed toes in the exercises that follow, we will specify "softly pointed" toes. This means that you should point your toes in a way that produces no sensation of tightness in your foot. You should just feel the sensation of stretching at the top of your foot. Don't curl your toes over at all.

The other foot position that's important in the Pilates Method is "flexed." This can be thought of as the opposite of pointed. When your feet are pointed, your toes are the part of you farthest from your head. When your feet are flexed, your heels should be farther from your head than your toes. You can accomplish this by simultaneously pushing your heels out away from you as far as they'll go and bending the top of your foot back, as if you were trying to touch your knee with your toes.

In flexing, as in pointing your toes, you don't want to tighten your foot and leg muscles to the point of cramping them. Concentrate on stretching out with your heel; then pull the top of your foot back as far as you can without straining.

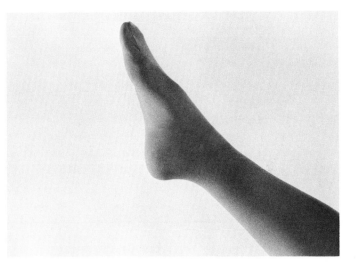

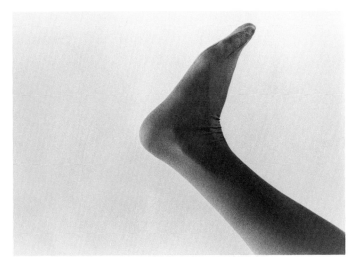

SITTING UP OUT OF YOUR HIPS

Sit facing a mirror. If you're sitting on the floor or a mat, your knees should be comfortably bent.

Visualize a string attached to the middle of your breastbone, running up to the ceiling at an angle just great enough so that it misses your chin. Someone is pulling up on that string, lifting your chest.

As your chest lifts, your back may be arching. This is not what we want, so release the string for a moment and visualize a pole that starts at the base of your spine and runs up through your spine and neck and out the top of your head. Make sure your spine is as straight as that pole. Now simultaneously visualize your chest lifted by the string and your head sliding as far up the pole as it can go.

You should be sitting much straighter than you were. A lot of the change in your position should have come in the area between your hipbones and your navel. Lift higher, paying

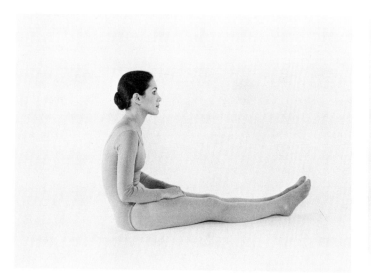

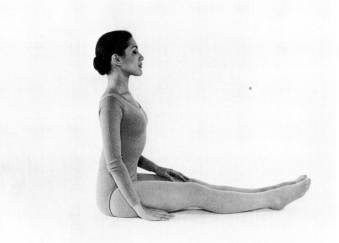

special attention to that area. Feel the sensation of your body growing taller, rising up from your hips.

This is what we mean by "sitting up out of your hips." Even with your chest pulled up and your head sliding up an imaginary pole so that your back is not arched, there is an extra bit of straightness and uprightness that comes from lifting the lowest part of your abdomen, as if you were stretching your navel away from your hips. To get this lift, it helps to pull your navel in toward your spine and make your center as firm as you can.

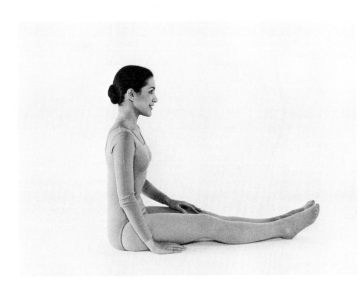

CHIN ON CHEST

Keeping your back straight, rotate your head so your chin moves toward your throat. Feel the pull at the back of your neck?

Relax these muscles at the back of your neck and move your chin toward your chest. Your neck should feel as if it is lengthening, and the pulling sensation should move down toward your back.

Many Pilates exercises require that you put your head in a position which Joe called "chin on chest."

It is a position which stretches the back of your neck and your spine, and it strengthens the muscles in your neck. When you are on your back, it helps you keep your spine anchored to the mat. In exercises in which you roll up and down from the mat, it helps you focus on your center. For some movements, it is a precaution against injury.

It's important that you do more than merely rotate your head forward. The idea is to lengthen your neck and feel the weight of your head pulling toward your center. Really reach for your chest with your chin. You won't make it, of course, but the attempt is what counts. Remember to relax those muscles at the back of your neck; imagine your neck growing longer as you reach for your sternum with the point of your chin.

At the beginning you may find this tiring, especially when you are on your back. Don't strain. As time passes, you will be able to hold your chin on your chest for longer periods of time.

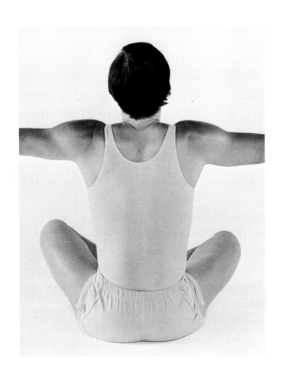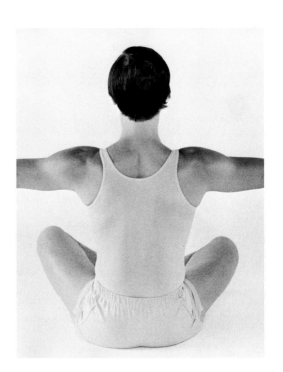

PINCHED BUTTOCKS

Next to the belly bulge, hip spread must be the most disliked visual symptom of lack of tone and fitness. And a chief culprit in hip spread is flaccid gluteal muscles. Buttocks, that is. Bottom. Bum. Or, as some would have it, buns.

Besides looking awful in a swimsuit or pants, bottom softness is also implicated in poor posture and an ungraceful stride. We would all be better off without it. To cure it, many exercise programs prescribe incessant repetitions of large, strenuous motions of the legs. But there is a small motion, almost no motion at all, that in the long run is much more effective. It is an integral part of many of the Pilates movements, and it's something you can do any time—waiting in line, or while you're cooking dinner, or on the beach.

You can learn to do this best if you are standing, though it's something you can do lying on your stomach or even on your back. In time, you'll be able to do it when you're sitting down.

To produce the effect we want, imagine a dime between your buttocks. Now squeeze your buttocks together so they pinch the dime between them. If you are standing up, your thighs should turn slightly outward when you do this, and the front of your pelvis should tilt upward.

Most important is the feeling of pressing your buttocks together and tightening them. Practice holding that dime in place until you are sure you are familiar with the sensation of what we will call "pinching your buttocks," or "pinching your bottom."

STRETCHING

In the spirit of "moving smoothly outward from a firm center," you will frequently be concerned with extending your arms and legs as much as possible.

The most common reaction to the instructions "straight arms" and "straight legs" is a tensing up that involves locking the elbows or knees. This is never useful; it tends to interfere with free motion and it can produce a kind of reverse bending of the arms or legs called "hyperextension." Combined with certain movements, it can lead to injury.

When we use the terms "straight arms" and "straight legs," we mean only "straight," not "locked."

If it is necessary in a movement for you to try for maximum extension of your arms or legs, we will ask you to "stretch your arms (long) out of your shoulders," or to "stretch your toes (or feet) (long) out of your hips."

To see what we mean by this, extend your arm straight in front of you. Do not lock your elbow. Visualize someone taking hold of your fingertips. (Better still, have someone actually do it.) Now, have your real or imagined partner gradually pull on your fingers. Hold your shoulder in place, but don't resist the pull. You should feel a stretching sensation that runs the whole length of your arm and focuses in your shoulder.

Now extend your arm straight up over your shoulder. Imagine your fingertips being pulled up to the ceiling by some invisible force. Again feel the uniform stretching throughout your arm and the sensation of the arm pulling away from the shoulder.

Lie down with your legs straight and together. Point your toes softly. Imagine someone pulling on them. Get the same feeling in your leg that you've just had in your arm. The whole leg stretches, from toes to hip, as if your toes were pulling your leg away from the hip joint.

While you're lying there, do one more experiment: put your arms straight out behind (over) your head. Now simultaneously (1) stretch your arms long out of your shoulders and (2) reach your toes as far from your hips as you can, stretching out of your hips. Imagine that you are on the rack, or that teams of horses are pulling in opposite directions on ropes attached to your feet and fingers. (Or think of a more pleasant image—for instance, two teams of handsome men or beautiful women playing tug of war, with you as the prize.) You are a string on a guitar or a violin, and the master is turning the key, pulling you taut. Feel the stretch in your limbs. Feel it especially in your shoulders and hips. This is what we mean by "stretch long and thin."

ONE VERTEBRA AT A TIME

Joe Pilates didn't like to see people make abrupt motions with their backs, especially with their backs straight. One of the earliest guiding principles of his method was that one should move the torso up and down from the mat in a smooth and gradual way.

"In coming up and going down," Joe said, "roll your spine exactly like a wheel. Vertebra by vertebra try to roll and unroll."

This principle has its most important application in the Pilates Method movements that more or less resemble the gym-class exercise called a "sit-up." The idea is always to roll up gradually, lifting one vertebra off the mat at a time, at no point levering yourself up the way you would in a sit-up. Roll, as Joe said, exactly like a wheel.

The same thing holds for letting your torso down onto the mat. Visualize your spine as a wheel with vertebrae attached to its rim, and roll down, *one vertebra at a time.*

This will not be easy at first, but it is a principle of cardinal importance. If you can't roll up all the way, roll up only as far as you can, and then use your arms to push or pull your body the rest of the way. Don't roll part-way up and jerk up the rest of the way.

The same holds for rolling down. Roll down as far as you can, concentrating on doing it one vertebra at a time. (Pinching your buttocks very tight will help.) When you can roll no farther, put your hands on the mat and lower yourself the rest of the way.

Rolling up and down one vertebra at a time helps make your back flexible, and it also helps you avoid the kind of abrupt motion that can cause injury.

Finding Your Body

Life is a process of constant change, one that requires constant learning. So it is with our bodies as well as our intellects.

In this chapter you have begun to find your body, and you have become familiar with some of the things that will be asked of it in the pages that follow. As you progress with the Pilates Method, your body's shape and capabilities will change; some of the changes may surprise you, but you will always be aware of them. Once you are truly embarked on a course that involves regular sessions of Pilates exercises, you will discover that you are always finding your body and—on new levels, with new depth and insight.

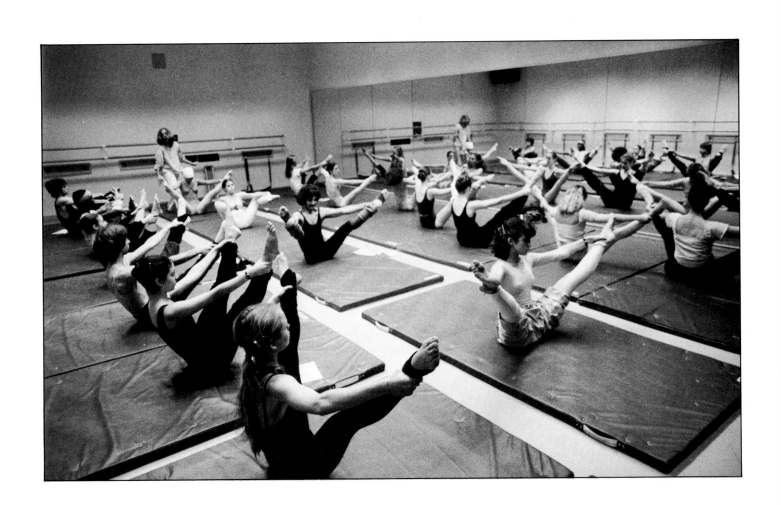

CHAPTER FIVE

First Steps

There Is No Free Lunch

Your body is an intricate mechanism—far more complicated than, say, your car. If you haven't been giving your body the regular tuning it needs, you can't expect to get it into proper operating condition without doing some work.

The Pilates Method will get you into shape without your having to endure the most unpleasant aspects of other forms of physical conditioning, and it is considerably more efficient, more effective, and more thorough than any other method, but it is not magic. To get the full advantage of its benefits, you have to make a commitment to it.

Progress by Stages

You may find, at first, that it is difficult even to come close to the proper form of the movement you are working on. (For instance, if the instructions say, "roll your back all the way up

off the mat," you may only be able to get your head and the tops of your shoulders up off the mat when you first try the movement.) That's all right. Just keep at it: concentrating, getting the breathing to work for you, making sure that you do carefully the things you can do. As time passes, your body will be stretched and toned, and you will be able to do more and more.

Bear in mind that the method is making you use muscles that you may have been neglecting for years, even if you've done other kinds of exercises in the recent past. At the beginning, some of the movements may seem strenuous. The tightening, lifting, and stretching required by the Pilates movements is not something most of us have experience with. So you may strain at first, and you may sometimes find yourself huffing and puffing. These are signs that you are working too hard or that you haven't got the parts of the movement properly coordinated. You may even (heaven forbid) be holding your breath.

With continued attention and practice, this should pass. In the meantime, you can take comfort from the fact that you're in good company. Joe Pilates used to comment that most professional athletes couldn't do his exercises properly when they started.

Even in the earliest learning stages, a session of Pilates exercises will be refreshing and it will work changes in your body. As the rudiments of each motion become second nature, you can concentrate on the fine points and on how the successive movements complement and flow into each other. Each session will become smoother, more of a whole. Where there was tension, there will now be relaxation. And the changes in your body, your breathing, your posture will become more noticeable.

Learning for Now . . . and for Always

Follow the program as we've outlined it. Start with only a few movements. Pay strict attention to the way you do them.

Like all of us when we are first exposed to the Pilates Method, you have almost certainly accumulated a lot of bad exercise habits over the years. It's vital that you begin to break them and learn the right approach. It's worth taking a little extra time and effort moving gradually into the Pilates Method. If you make it a part of yourself, its effects will carry over into everyting you do, and it will stand you in good stead the rest of your life.

Before You Begin

While the Pilates Method will help you discover and correct weaknesses and imbalances you never knew you had, there are some preliminary inquiries you should make before you start.

Before you begin this or any other new program of exercise, you should consult a doctor.

When people come to the Pilates Studio (some of them sent by their physicians) great care is taken to determine their individual physical limitations and to custom-design an introductory program of exercise for them if one seems indicated. We can't do that for you. All we can do is set out the standard program and remind you not to do anything that feels like it is a strain, or anything that causes pain. But this may not be enough. Your doctor is the person best able to tell if there is any kind of movement or exertion that is likely to prove troublesome to you, and your doctor is also the person to ask how your heart will react to your learning the Pilates Method. These questions are especially important if you have not been getting some regular form of exercise recently.

Learning a New Movement

Before you begin to do a new movement, read the instructions through. *Out loud. Twice.*

As you read each instruction, refer to the pictures and try to visualize the motion in your mind. You will do better at this the second time than the first. It may help you to go through some of the motions, trying out any parts that may seem unclear to you or difficult to coordinate, to get a kinetic sense of the exercise, so that when you actually begin to do it, your body will be familiar with the movements it has to make. Also, consider how the rhythm of breathing fits in naturally with the motions; it should actually help you to move.

Read all the way to the end of the instructions each time. Don't just skim through for the parts you think are the minimum necessary to get a reasonable approximation of the pictures. *All of the instructions are important.*

Remember—the goal is to perform each movement with ultimate control, coordination, and precision. In order to do an exercise correctly, you must be fully familiar with the instructions for movement and breathing and aware of the exercise's checkpoints for concentration. Even when you think you know how to do a given exercise, you will always be able to profit from a review of its instructions.

Getting Away with It

One of the things that virtually every other method of physical conditioning encourages is an attitude of—okay, I'm going to get this done any old way, just as long as I get through it. (If only I can do twenty of these damn things, then I can stop with a clear conscience.)

But the immediate goal in the Pilates Method is never to do a certain number of exercises, or a certain exercise a large number of times. The most basic rule is always—one properly done movement is worth any number of sloppy ones.

If you are tired, rushed, hung over, or otherwise out of sorts, don't try to get through your whole program of movements doing each one halfheartedly. Instead, do just one movement, or two, or three—as many as you can—with total concentration. And don't decide how many that is before you start. Do them one at a time, as well as possible, until you feel you should stop. *But do at least one.*

Of course, you are the only person who can know if you're *really* concentrating, if you're really trying to do each movement *as well as you possibly can at the time.* If you let yourself get away with less than your best, you are the one who loses out.

An Important Note:

Doing your best is a concept that has nothing to do with competition. You are not competing with someone else. You are not even competing with what you did last time, or any other time. You are not trying to reach some arbitrary goal you set for yourself in advance. What you are doing is putting your total attention and effort into executing each motion with the greatest degree of control and precision and with the best coordination of breathing and movement you are capable of at the time you are doing it.

Using a Mirror

If you can arrange it comfortably, going through all or part of your Pilates session in front of a mirror can be very useful.

Pay careful attention to how your body feels and how it looks. Is your leg really straight when you think it is? Reach with heel or toes to straighten it more. It will feel different. How?

Are you sitting up out of your hips as tall as possible? Is your back arched? Can you sit taller without arching your back?

Don't just admire yourself—measure your actual performance against the instructions for each movement, and especially against the checkpoints.

Partnership

It's good to exercise with someone else, at least once in a while. Even though when you're exercising alone you concentrate as hard as you can on everything you're doing, you can't always tell exactly how your body is moving. Using a mirror is not the whole answer to this problem, if only because looking in a mirror can interfere with doing some of the exercises properly.

But if you have a friend (or spouse, or lover) exercising with you now and then, it can be very beneficial for both of you.

Try this: as you're doing an exercise, let your partner read the instructions to you. *Listen carefully,* letting the words guide you through a mental inventory of your body. Are you following the instructions completely? Your partner should watch you carefully, and the second time you do the exercise, your partner should read the hints and checkpoints that follow the exercise's instructions. Again, listen carefully and relate what you are hearing to what you are doing. The third time, your partner should point out anything you are doing that is inconsistent with the instructions. This is where a second point of view is especially helpful.

Bear in mind that this is not meant to be criticism. No one ever performs a difficult physical movement perfectly every time. Not an athlete. Not a dancer. In the case of the Pilates Method, long experience has shown that hearing the words spoken can be a powerful aid to concentration. When you work with a partner, it is for your benefit, and it will have an important positive effect on you. If your partner points out ways in which you can do the exercises more accurately, you are not being scolded; rather, you are being given information useful for determining whether you are producing the results you intend to. (Of course, your partner should also understand the purpose of the corrections and make them in that spirit.)

Doing the exercises with a partner is best if you are both participating, alternately exercising and reading and watching for each other. But even someone whose exposure to the Pilates Method is limited to reading for you and watching you exercise can be very helpful.

For the Non-exercising Partner:

In addition to making verbal corrections, it can help to touch your partner gently on the place you want to call attention to. If one of your partner's shoulders is hunched up, for instance, you might combine a verbal correction with a light touch on the muscle that joins shoulder to neck on that side. Sometimes it's hard for the person doing the movement to isolate a muscle that needs to be tightened or relaxed, and having the muscle touched singles it out and focuses the exerciser's attention on it.

Make a Tape

Another way to give yourself a reminder of what you're doing while you're doing it is to read the instructions for the exercises in your program into a tape recorder. You can play the tape back to yourself as you go through your session. Better still—when you're working with a partner, record your partner's instructions and comments. In either case, you'll need to re-record the tape frequently if you are going to keep up with your own progress.

A precaution: because the state of your body will vary from day to day, the inflexibility of instructions recorded on tape may result in your sometimes being pressed to go faster or slower than you would if you found your own pace. This can be especially troublesome if it tends to speed you up significantly beyond what would be comfortable for you on a given day.

Equipment

Very little specialized equipment is required to do the Pilates Method mat work. The only absolutely essential item is a padded surface you can lie on.

NEVER EXERCISE ON THE BARE FLOOR WITHOUT PROPER PADDING. YOU WILL HURT YOUR SPINE.

A well-padded rug may be enough to cushion your movements, but a standard exercise mat (the kind you see in a gym) is much better. There are commercially available exercise boards (usually intended mostly for sit-ups, or for certain kinds of weightlifting); these vary in hardness, and some may be too hard. If you are going to buy one, try it out first. If you can't take it home with full return privileges, do some exercises on it in the store. If that isn't possible or practical, don't buy it. The Pilates Method involves many movements in which your back rolls on the mat. Your spine is too valuable to entrust to a mat that does not protect it well enough.

A Homemade Mat:

Fold a standard medium-weight wool or synthetic blanket *twice* in half the long way to make four layers of cloth. You will have a pad six or so feet long and more than a foot wide. This should be ideal, but since blankets vary in thickness and resilience, you should test it the way you would test a store-bought exercise mat.

There are other possibilities, such as a foam-rubber cushion, a partially inflated air mattress or a sleeping bag, but each of these has its drawbacks. Whatever you use, it must provide sufficient padding to keep you from bruising your spine, and it must also be steady and secure, so that it forms a solid base for your movements. If it shifts or changes shape during an exercise, it could cause discomfort or even injury; it will certainly interfere with your doing the exercise properly.

Although Joe Pilates did design some exercises to be done in bed (and a special bed for doing the exercises) we do not recommend that you do the exercises in this book while you are in bed.

For a few of the exercises it may be useful to have a heavy piece of furniture to put your feet under, so that they will be held close to the floor. Dressers are frequently good for this. (If there's no space under the frame to put your feet, pull out the bottom drawer just far enough to brace your toes under it.) You might also use a solid, low-bottomed chair.

If you are using a store-bought or homemade exercise mat with a wooden base, you can attach a length of cloth or leather strap to one end of it to brace your feet. This is how the mats at the Pilates Studio work. An old length of belt, especially a webbed cloth belt, is ideal. The ends of the strap should be attached to the board at least a foot apart, with just enough slack so that you can get your feet comfortably under the strap.

What to Wear

In choosing clothes to exercise in, pick something that will not bind or restrict your movement and does not have anything that will hinder your circulation (a tight belt, for instance). For women, the best choice is a leotard, with or without tights; for men, a T-shirt or tank top worn with comfortable shorts or swimming trunks and an athletic supporter.

No Strain, No Pain

Don't force yourself into positions that your body doesn't want to take. Don't strain to complete any movement past the point where it begins to create discomfort. The idea is to build your body, not to break it down.

We're not saying you should take it easy or that you shouldn't exert yourself. By all means, as you become familiar with the method and as your program of exercise expands, work up a sweat. Do every movement to the maximum extent of your ability. Press to your limits. Don't slack off. But don't go beyond your ability, and don't do any movement past the point at which you have control of what your body is doing. It is a sure path to injury.

When to Exercise

Any time at all.

There are some obvious cautions: not right after eating, not when you're sick; not when you're seriously fatigued from other activity or severe lack of sleep (although this caution has to be balanced with the fact that a short Pilates session can be a real waker-up); not when you've been drinking heavily or using drugs that will affect your heart or blood pressure, or your judgment.

People have different inclinations about when to exercise. Our best advice is: follow your own. We like to do our sessions in the morning, to get us going, but we also do some exercises during the day, as refreshers (see Chapter Nine), and in the evening, to counteract the effects of the day's work. Some Pilates regulars are scandalized by the very notion of morning exercise, but they do a full session every day after work. Not only does it refresh them, but it helps them throw off the day's tensions and frustrations, so that they can enjoy their evening.

Actor Tony Roberts has an interesting schedule. "I'll do five minutes of the mat work in the morning, and then more in the evening. There are some times when I get up in the middle of the night. I'll do a few minutes of mat work and find myself relaxed and feeling better."

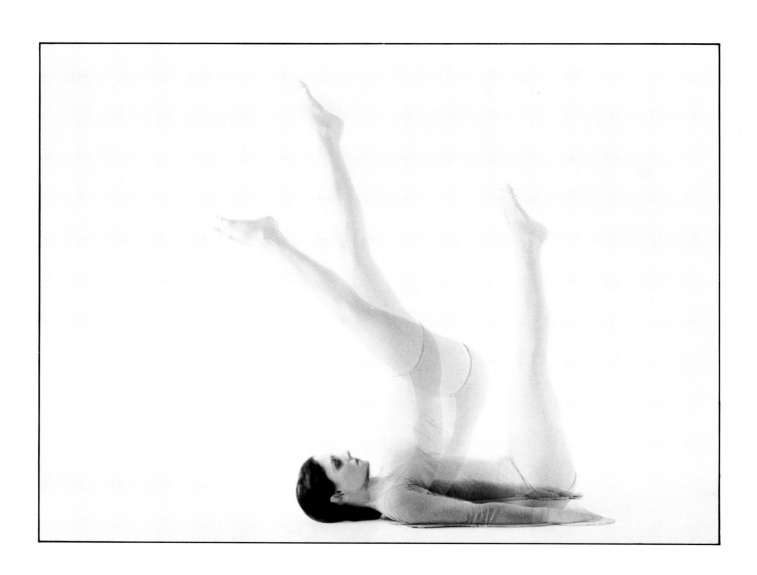

CHAPTER SIX

On Your Way

In this chapter, you'll find a starter program of exercises balanced and organized to involve a full complement of muscles and help you become familiar with the Pilates Method.

There are ten exercises (the names, like the exercises, are the work of Joe Pilates):

THE HUNDRED	DOUBLE-LEG STRETCH
ROLL-UP	SPINE STRETCH
LEG CIRCLES	SAW
ROLLING	SIDE KICK
SINGLE-LEG STRETCH	SEAL

You should do these in the order in which they appear in the book, whether you do all ten or fewer.

At the beginning, you should do *no more than five*. The right ones to start with are:

THE HUNDRED
ROLL-UP
SINGLE-LEG STRETCH
SPINE STRETCH
SEAL

Instructions for these exercises are on pages 50, 52, 58, 62, and 68.

We recommend that you do these first five exercises every day to begin with. It won't take long, and the early continuity is an important aid to learning the rudiments of the method.

In any case, try not to let a day go by without doing *at least one* of the exercises.

After two weeks, if you feel you are beginning to master the first five exercises, increase your program gradually to ten. *Do not add more than one new movement a session.*

Keep trying to do at least one exercise every day. Do your entire program three times a week or more.

Do not progress past this stage until you have been doing all ten exercises regularly for at least a dozen sessions.

There is no reason to hurry on to add new movements. There is plenty to learn and much to be gained in these first ten.

A WORD ABOUT THE INSTRUCTIONS AND THE PICTURES

The exercise instructions you'll find in the following pages are likely to look different from the ones you've seen before.

At first glance the instructions may seem long and complicated. As you use them, you'll find that their precision—one of the basic Pilates principles—plays a large part in the unique value of the method.

The photographs are intended to help you understand the instructions quickly, completely, and accurately. When you are more experienced in the method, they can be used as a quick reference and memory refresher.

However, the photographs do not give you enough information to do the exercises without reading the instructions.

In particular, not all of the photographs show the exercises carried to the extreme point of movement. Some people start out more limber than others, or stronger. Control and precision are more important than doing an exercise to the furthest point described in the instructions. The very fact that at first you will not be able to do the movements completely adds to the amount of change and development you can experience with the Pilates Method. There is always room for improvement.

If the pictures and the instructions aren't in exact agreement on the limits of a movement, you should use the instructions as your ultimate authority. If you can do better than the pictures, go ahead. But whatever the instructions say, never force a movement past the point of strain.

In Pursuit of the Flatteringly Flat Belly

One of the most familiar exercises is the ordinary sit-up, the standard gym-class exercise for what are usually called the "stomach muscles." With slight variations, sit-ups appear in virtually every program of physical conditioning.

Most people, unaware of the myriad benefits of firming the center of their bodies, have but one thing in mind when they do their sit-ups: that most desired and most elusive of physical characteristics, the flat belly.

Even for simple fitness, the ordinary sit-up isn't much good at its job. It's a lot more likely to involve the hip-flexor muscles than the abdominal muscles. Even the few fitness-book exercises that actually manage to involve the abdominal muscles are only minimally helpful to those in search of a firm, fit, and *flat* abdomen. Because of the motions involved, and because of the way the exercises are described, they all encourage you *to stick your stomach out* while you're doing them!

The Pilates Method, on the other hand, trains you to hold these muscles in a *flat* or pulled-in position. And, as you progress, this training won't end when you're through exercising— it will carry over into the way you hold your abdominal muscles all day long.

Largely because of the concept of the strong center, almost all the Pilates movements involve the abdomen, all the way down to the hard to reach muscles at the hip line. By providing a constant and varied emphasis on this area, the Pilates Method can give you firmer abdominal muscles, better posture, and a *much flatter* belly.

You have already begun to develop your center, and to concentrate on keeping your belly flat, by doing The Hundred. The next exercise—the Roll-Up—will take you farther in that direction.

THE HUNDRED

Always start with The Hundred to stimulate your circulation and breathing.

Anchoring

1. Lie flat on your back with your arms by your sides, palms down.
2. Anchor yourself in place by pressing your spine to the mat. Try to make your navel touch your spine (but don't suck in your stomach or hold your breath—think of a heavy weight pressing down your middle).

Position

3. Bend your knees and bring them to your chest, pressing your spine closer to the mat. Straighten your legs, keeping them together, to about a right angle with the floor.
4. Chin on chest.
5. With your legs straight and your toes softly pointed, lower your legs until your spine begins to arch off the mat. Stop. Press your spine down, raising your legs slightly if necessary.
6. Lift your hands about six inches off the mat next to your body, palms down, with your arms and wrists straight, reaching away from your shoulders with your fingertips.

Movement

7. Pump your arms up and down rapidly a few inches (toward the ceiling and toward the mat) in short, vigorous motions for five counts.

Continue in groups of five for up to one hundred pumps.

Breathing

Breathe IN for five pumping motions.
OUT for five pumping motions.
If you do a hundred, you will take ten deep breaths.

Hints for Beginners

1. One hundred pumping motions may be tiring at first. Start with twenty (two complete deep breaths) and work up to a hundred by adding five at a time.
2. If your neck muscles get tired, lower your head to the mat for a few pumping motions, then raise it again if you can.

3. If your legs tend to sink as you do The Hundred, raise them higher, instead.

4. Eventually, your toes should be on a line with your eyes. For now, lower them only as far as you can while keeping your spine pressed flat to the mat.

Checkpoints

1. Keep yourself firmly anchored to the mat.

2. Navel to spine.

3. Eyes on your stomach. Watch to make sure it doesn't bulge.

4. Empty your lungs completely with each breath.

5. Don't hunch your shoulders. Reach with your fingertips.

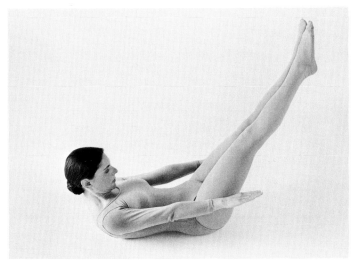

ROLL-UP

You will need a bar about a yard long. A broomstick will do, a yardstick, or an umbrella. If you don't have something around, pretend you have one in your hands as you do the movement.

Anchoring and Position

1. Lie flat on your back. Legs together, feet flexed.
2. Holding the bar in both hands, put your hands on the mat over your head, arms straight.
3. Spine to mat. Navel to spine.
4. Stretch long and thin from your hands to your heels.

Movement

5. Reaching out of your shoulders as if someone were pulling on the bar, lift your arms from the mat. Lift your head, too, keeping your ears between your arms.
6. Roll up by bringing your head between your upraised arms as if you were looking through a window.
7. Keep your arms moving, imagining someone pulling on the bar until your hands are aimed at a point just above and beyond your feet. At the same time, continue to roll up, lifting one vertebra at a time off the mat. Let your hands pull you forward until you can go no farther. Your chin is on your chest, your heels pushing away from your hips. Navel to spine.

8. Reverse the movement, rolling back down one vertebra at a time. Pinch your buttocks tight and push your heels away from your hips, while visualizing someone holding the bar, lowering you gently to the mat.
9. Keep your chin on your chest and navel pressed toward your spine.
10. When your shoulderblades reach the mat, start to bring your arms overhead, reaching out, and lower your head, so that you return to Position.

Do up to five Roll-Ups. Two are enough to start with.

Breathing

Breathe IN as you roll up, until you're sitting up.
OUT as you reach forward.
IN beginning to roll back.
OUT as you approach the mat.

Hints for Beginners

1. Hook your feet under a piece of furniture to help anchor yourself.
2. Reaching forward, bend your knees a little. When you can't reach any farther, try to straighten your legs.
3. If at first you can't roll up, just bring your arms around

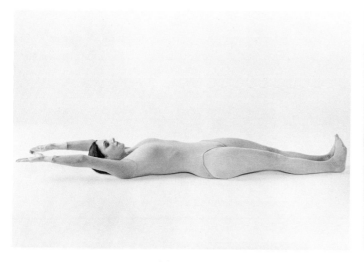

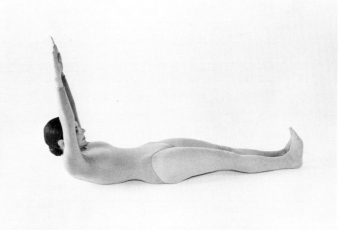

and reach for your toes with the bar. Try to lift one or two vertebrae off the mat. Then help yourself into a sitting position and stretch forward with the bar, keeping your chin on your chest.

4. Your partner can actually pull on the bar (if you have a partner). Don't pull too hard: pull evenly and gradually. Feel the resistance. Relax.

Checkpoints

1. Keep your stomach *flat*.
2. Chin on chest as you roll up and roll down.
3. Push heels away from hips. Feet flexed.
4. One vertebra at a time.

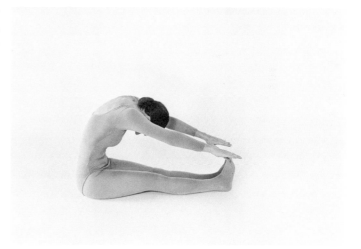

LEG CIRCLES

Anchoring

1. Lie flat on your back, arms by your sides, palms down, legs together.
2. Spine to mat. Navel to spine. Stretch your neck long.
3. Feel yourself anchored along your spine; press your palms into the mat. Do the same with the base of your skull.

Position

4. Raise your right leg as high as you can, keeping your spine anchored firmly to the mat.
5. Both legs are straight. You can either flex your feet or point them. It is good to alternate from time to time.

Movement

6. Make a circle with your leg—across your body, down toward the mat, out and up.
7. Hold for a moment. Think of stretching your leg toward your face (but don't bend your knee).
8. Do three to five circles, then reverse direction.

Each leg does three to five circles in each direction.

Breathing

Breathe OUT for the first half of the Leg Circle.

IN as you swing your leg back up.

Hints for Beginners

1. Start off with small Leg Circles, only a foot or so around, concentrating on keeping your back, neck and one leg pressed to the mat and motionless. Your goal is to make the circles larger as you become more proficient, always keeping yourself firmly anchored.
2. Before starting each group of circles, lie in Position and gently pull your raised leg toward you.
3. If you can't raise your leg straight off the mat, bend your knee to your chest and then push your foot into the air.

Checkpoints

1. Legs straight (especially the raised one).
2. Spine to mat.
3. Navel to spine. No stomach bulge.
4. Don't let your neck arch. Skull to mat and neck long.
5. Use your palms to keep from rocking side to side (press palms to mat).
6. Don't make your Leg Circles too large. Keep them controlled.

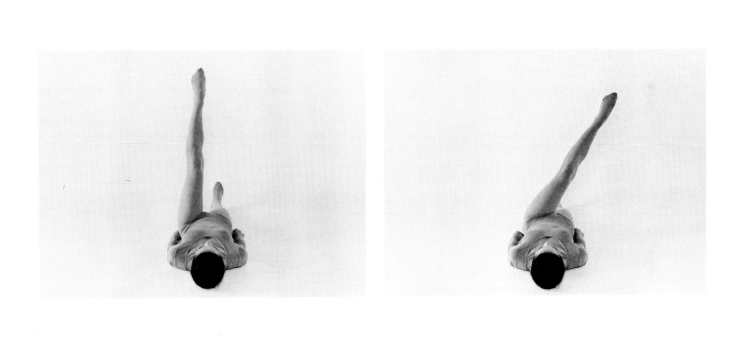

ROLLING (LIKE A BALL)

This is a relaxing exercise, a massage for the spine.

Position

1. Sit on the mat and bring your knees to your chest. (You should be near the end of the mat.)
2. Navel to spine. Round your back and wrap your arms around your legs. Grasp your right ankle with your left hand and your left wrist with your right hand.
3. Bring your heels close to your bottom and lower your chin to your chest. Tighten your arms around your legs.

Movement

4. Roll back like a ball until your bottom leaves the mat. Stay tight.
5. Pull down firmly on your legs with your arms to help you start rolling back up without uncurling.
6. Roll all the way up to Position.

Roll back and forth rhythmically eight to ten times.

Breathing

Breathe IN as you roll backward.

OUT as you roll up.

Hints for Beginners

1. Press your thighs to your chest and try to make yourself into a ball by curling your head toward your stomach.
2. Pull hard on your legs to come up.

Checkpoints

1. No stomach bulge!
2. Chin on chest.
3. Heels close to bottom.
4. Maintain control. Don't roll too far back.

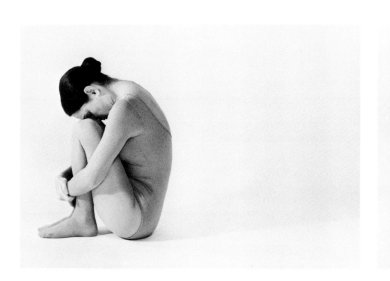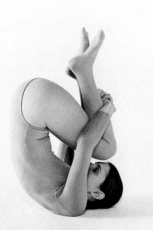

SINGLE-LEG STRETCH

Anchoring

1. Lie flat on your back. Anchor yourself by pressing your spine to the mat. Navel to spine.

Position

2. Your legs are stretched long and your toes softly pointed. Bring your right knee to your chest.
3. Grasp your ankle with your right hand and your knee with your left. Your elbows should be out from your body and raised.
4. Lift your head until your chin is on your chest. Focus on your center.
5. Raise your left foot off the mat just high enough to keep your back from arching, stretching from your hip to your toes.

Movement

6. Switch the positions of your legs—reaching long with the toes of your right foot as you bend your left knee close to your chest, grasping your knee with your right hand and your ankle with your left.
7. Pull the left leg as close to your chest as you can, while reaching as long as possible with your right foot.

Do five to eight stretches with each leg, alternating.

Breathing

Breathe IN for two leg stretches.
OUT for two.
Rhythm is essential.
Both inhalation and exhalation are *long* and *gradual*.
Be sure to force all the air from your lungs on the exhalation.

Hints for Beginners

1. To get your extended leg into Position, bring it to your chest, and then extend it into the air the way you did getting into Position for The Hundred. Remember not to lower it past the point where your back starts to arch off the mat.
2. At first, you may not be able to get your knee at all close to your chest. Don't strain or force it when you pull. You will loosen up gradually.
3. If you can't reach your ankle, grab your leg higher up, on the shin.
4. You may not be able to hold your head up for all the leg

stretches you do. Start by keeping your chin on your chest and your eyes on your navel for one pair of stretches, then lower your head to the mat. Build up gradually.

Checkpoints

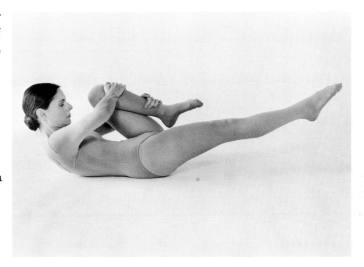

1. Toes pointed.
2. Watch your stomach! Don't let it bulge.
3. Your shoulders should be relaxed. Don't let them hunch up.
4. Keep the movement smooth and flowing.
5. Head forward. Chin on chest.

Ideally, your feet should almost skim the mat, with your foot at eye level when it is fully extended.

DOUBLE-LEG STRETCH

Anchoring

1. Lie flat on your back. Anchor yourself by pressing your spine to the mat. Navel to spine. Feet pointed softly.

Position

2. Bend both legs close to your chest. Grasp your shins and press your legs to your chest, forcing out all the air in your lungs.
3. Lift your head until your chin is on your chest. Focus on your firm center.

Movement

4. Extend *both* legs the way you extended one for the Single-Leg Stretch. Keep your legs together and your feet pointed.
5. At the same time, sweep your hands up toward the ceiling and over (behind) your head, keeping them shoulder width or closer, fingers reaching long.
6. At the end of the outward stretch, your legs are pulling out of your hips through your toes, while your fingers reach as far as possible, stretching out of your shoulders.

Think of yourself as long and thin, like a taut piece of string. Don't let your back arch.

7. Sweep your arms out to your sides, keeping them close to the mat, while bending your knees to return to Position.

Do up to five smooth, graceful stretches.

Breathing

Breathe IN as you stretch your arms and legs OUT.

OUT as you bring your legs and arms IN toward your chest.

Press your legs to your chest to force all the air from your lungs.

Hints for Beginners

1. Remember not to let your legs drop past the point where your back begins to arch off the mat.
2. Don't strain or force your legs to get them close to your chest.
3. You may not be able to hold your head up for very long, at first. Start by lifting your head as far as you can (chin on chest, if possible) for only one stretch-and-return.

Checkpoints

1. Keep your toes pointed.

2. Watch your stomach! No bulge. (If you can't see it, sense it. Pay attention to your navel.)

3. Your shoulders should be relaxed. Don't let them hunch up.

4. Keep the movement smooth and flowing.

5. Your arms should stretch long, fingers pointed, making a wide, graceful circle.

6. Keep your head forward (chin on chest) as much as you can.

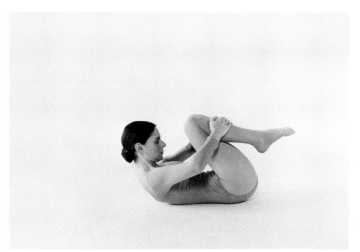 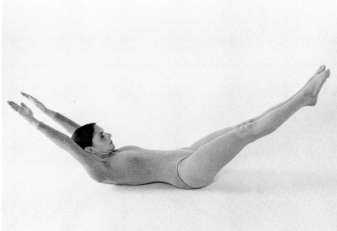

SPINE STRETCH

In spite of its name, this is basically a breathing exercise.

Anchoring and Position

1. Sit on the mat with your legs spread a little more than shoulder width.
2. Your toes should be flexed, your knees loose or slightly bent.
3. Anchor your buttocks to the mat. Sit up out of your hips.
4. Navel to spine.

Movement

5. Curl in and down. Aim the top of your head toward the center of your stomach.
6. At the same time, stretch forward with your hands, reaching past an imaginary line running between your feet.
7. While you are stretching outward and curling in, keep your navel attached to your spine.
8. When you can go no farther, pause and press knees toward the mat, reaching out with your toes and your fingers.

9. Return to Position by reversing the motion, always concentrating on keeping your head curled down, even as you sit up.

Do up to five stretches, paying particular attention to your breathing.

Breathing

Breathe IN when returning to Position.

OUT on the way down, concentrating on forcing the air from your lungs on the farthest point of your stretch.

Hints for Beginners

1. Don't spread your legs too far.
2. It's not necessary to get your legs straight at first or to stretch very far forward. Stop if you feel any discomfort.
3. Concentrate primarily on curling your head toward your navel and keeping your navel glued to your spine.
4. It's the breathing and coordination that are important.

Checkpoints

1. Don't hunch your shoulders or let them rise as you reach forward.

2. Navel to spine.

3. Force all the air from your lungs—one, two, three— while reaching and curling.

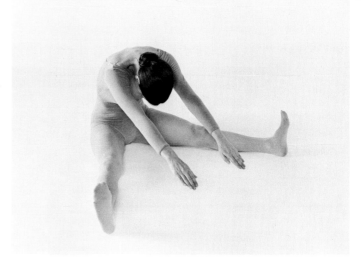

THE SAW

Anchoring

1. Sit on the mat with your legs spread a little more than shoulder width.
2. Legs straight, heels pushed out, feet flexed.
3. Your buttocks and heels are anchored firmly to the mat.

Position

4. Visualize a pole running from the base of your spine up through the top of your head. Slide your head up the pole as far as possible, sitting up out of your hips.
5. Raise your arms straight out at your sides, parallel to the floor, palms down, fingertips reaching outward.

Movement

6. Rotate your body, at the same time reaching *past* your left foot with your right hand, so that your pinky and the edge of your hand slide along the base of your little toe, as if you were sawing off your toes with the edge of your hand.
7. As your right hand reaches forward, stretch your left hand out behind you, raising it as high as possible.

8. Let your head follow your forward arm. Keep your buttocks to the mat.
9. Return to Position by reversing the motion of instructions 6, 7, and 8. Move smoothly and with control, sitting up out of your hips.
10. Reverse, sawing at your right toes with your left hand and stretching up and back with your right.

Repeat three to five times to each side.

Breathing

Start by breathing IN as you push your head up the pole.

Push the air gradually and steadily OUT of your lungs as you reach forward.

Breathe IN while returning to Position.

Hints for Beginners

1. If necessary, start with your knees slightly bent.
2. Don't worry about reaching your toes. It's more important to keep yourself firmly anchored and do the movement with control.

Checkpoints

1. Try not to bend your knees (or, if you are starting with bent knees, try not to bend them any more as you reach forward).

2. Do not let your hip rise as you reach forward.

3. Each time you return to Position, try to slide your head up that pole, sitting up out of your hips.

4. Don't hunch your shoulders.

5. Keep your navel glued to your spine.

6. Make sure your hand does not drop below the level of your toes.

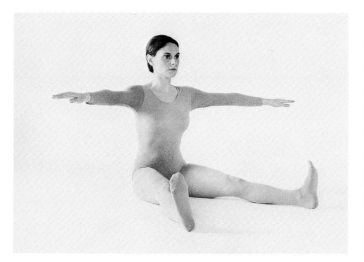
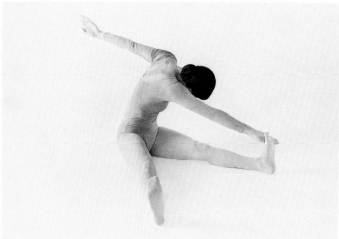

SIDE KICK

Anchoring and Position

1. Lie on your right side with your head resting on your raised right hand, your right elbow extended on a line with your body. You should try to be one straight line, tailbone to elbow.

2. Bend at the hips, so that your legs are still straight, but at an angle with your body, the left leg resting on the right.

3. Brace your left hand on the mat in front of your chest.

4. Anchor your entire body to the mat, from foot to elbow.

5. Your left hipbone should be directly above your right, your bottom foot lightly flexed.

6. Navel to spine. Concentrate on maintaining a firm center.

Movement

7. With your left (top) foot softly pointed, stretch the leg, reaching out of your hip. Your foot should be exactly at hip level.

8. Kick your left leg forward, keeping it at hip level over the mat. The kick is in two motions—the first, a long sweeping kick as "high" (toward your face) as you can comfortably go. The second part is a little bounce im-

mediately following the first, pushing the foot a little farther.

9. Sweep your leg back, your foot still lightly pointed, still at hip level, reaching out of your hip, kicking as far backward as you can (past your anchored leg). Again there is a second, bouncing, extra kick.

10. Immediately start a new kick forward.

11. Note especially: throughout, keep yourself anchored firmly and *try not to move your torso or hips.*

Do up to five kicks, then turn over and do the same number on the other side.

Breathing

Breathe IN as you kick forward.

OUT as you kick back.

Hints for Beginners

1. Don't kick too far up or too far back, or you will lose your Position.

2. Use your hand on the mat to help stay motionless except for your kicking leg.

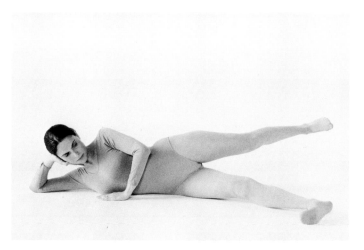

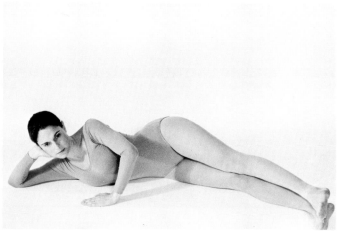

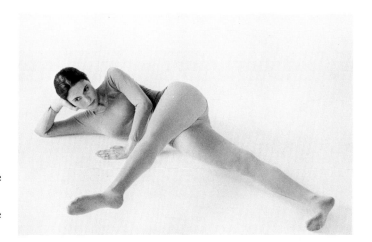

Checkpoints

1. Keep your anchor firm and motionless.
2. Navel to spine. Very firm center.
3. Make sure the top hipbone stays directly over the anchored one.
4. Make sure your kicking leg stays at hip level above the mat.

SEAL

Position

1. Sit with your feet on the mat, your soles pressed together.
2. Bring your arms to your center and reach through the space between your knees, bringing your hands outside your ankles and wrapping them around your feet.
3. Navel to spine.
4. Chin on chest.

Movement

5. Roll smoothly onto your back; go far enough back to lift your seat from the mat and shift your weight onto your shoulderblades.
6. Immediately roll forward until your feet touch the mat again, or as far as you can go.

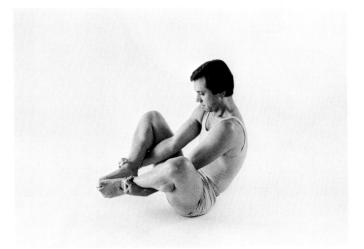
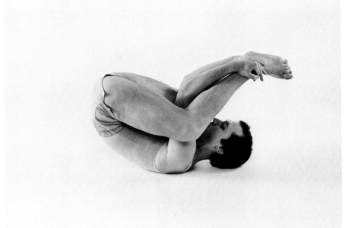

Breathing

Breathe OUT as you roll back.

IN as you roll up.

Hints for Beginners

1. If you can't press your soles together, start by pressing the inside edges of your feet together, then roll the soles toward each other as far as they will go. (Your knees, of course, will be spread wide.)

2. Don't roll too far back, at first.

3. The essential ingredient of the Seal is—don't relax your center. Most of the motive force comes from your abdomen.

Checkpoints

1. Chin on chest.

2. Smooth motion back and forth.

3. Navel to spine. Don't let your stomach bulge!

FLOWING MOTION

Now that you have mastered the introductory sequence of exercises, you can begin to apply the basic principles of the Pilates Method to the spaces between the exercises. Try to make *every movement* smooth and flowing, done with control and precision and without wasted motion, from one end of your session to the other. Progress gracefully from the end of one exercise to the beginning of the next. Adding a new exercise is like adding a new step to a dance routine—each movement should flow smoothly into the one that follows it.

NOTHING TO IT?

If you find the early stages easy, don't press ahead too quickly. It is likely to be a sign that you aren't doing the movements with full concentration and control. Try harder. Pay special attention to the checkpoints.

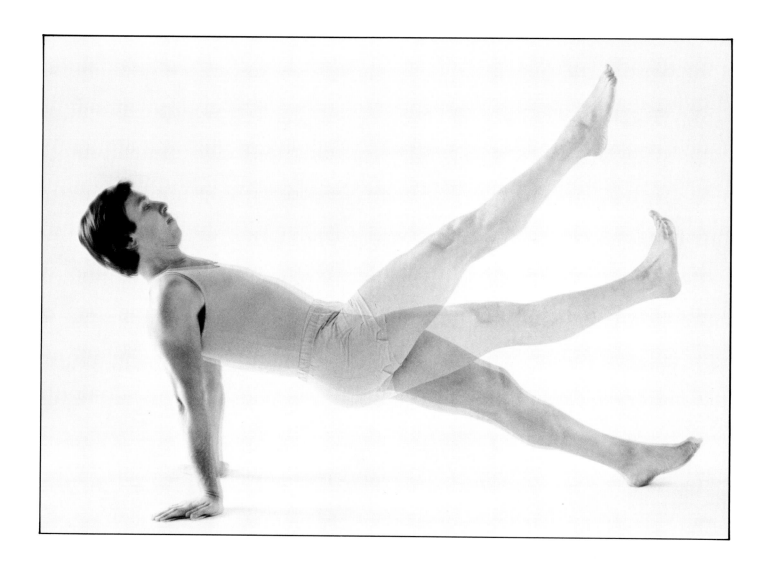

CHAPTER SEVEN

Onward to the Full Program

This chapter gives instructions for thirty-two exercises, plus variations. The whole group, in the order they're presented here, is the full Pilates Method mat-work program. Both the details of the exercises and the order they appear in are important.

When you have become thoroughly familiar with the ten exercises in Chapter Six you can begin to add new movements to your program.

As we've said, there's no need to progress quickly to a dozen or fifteen or twenty exercises; you don't have to feel you're missing out if you haven't mastered the whole program. You can be admirably stretched and toned and develop strength and grace and improved posture, even if over a considerable period of time you simply do regular sessions of the Chapter Six movements, as long as you do them with total concentration, increasing control and precision, and thorough attention to keeping your movements smooth and flowing and coor-dinated with your breathing. And if you're not doing them that way, you won't get much increased benefit from adding new ones, anyway. Remember, how you do things is more important than what you do.

As with the Chapter Six exercises, you should *add no more than one new movement a session*. Take your time with each new exercise. After a few sessions, it will integrate itself into your program.

Expanding Your Program

You shouldn't pick new movements from the full program haphazardly. There is a definite progression to follow. You'll find it, in five separate levels, in the pages that follow.

Level 1

These are the movements you are already familiar with. However, in some cases the instructions given here are more advanced than those in Chapter Six.

When you've mastered these, move on to Level 2.

Level 2

Add these movements, one at a time, in the order they're given. Each movement fits into its proper position relative to the whole program.

Substitute Rolling II for Rolling I and Seal II for Seal I any time it feels comfortable.

Level 3

Add these movements, one at a time, in this order, putting them in their proper place relative to the whole program.

		page
1.	CORKSCREW I	92
2.	DOUBLE-LEG KICK	106
3.	SPINE TWIST	118
4.	TEASER I	128
5.	HIP CIRCLES	134
6.	SWIMMING	145
7.	TEASER II	130

Substitute Open-Leg Rocker II for Open-Leg Rocker I and Corkscrew II for Corkscrew I any time it feels comfortable.

Level 4

Add these exercises, in this order, one at a time, in their proper place relative to the whole program.

		page
1.	ROLL-OVER	78
2.	SIDE KICK LIFT	127
3.	LEG-PULL FRONT	136
4.	LEG-PULL	138
5.	TWIST I	140
6.	CONTROL BALANCE	152

Whenever you're ready, substitute Corkscrew III for Corkscrew II, Swan Dive II for Swan Dive I, and Teaser III for both Teaser I and Teaser II.

These are advanced exercises. They require a high level of control.

Level 5   **BE PREPARED**

Add these exercises, one at a time, in any order that appeals to you, but keep them in their proper places relative to the full program.

These are advanced exercises. They require a high level of control.

Remember—before you do a new movement, read the instructions through at least twice, paying attention to what you are reading and thinking about it. Visualize the movement.

THE HUNDRED

Anchoring

1. Lie on your back with your arms by your sides. Legs straight, toes softly pointed.
2. Spine to mat. Navel to spine.

Position

3. Chin on chest.
4. Lift your straight legs off the mat and then lower them until your spine begins to arch off the mat. Stop. Press your spine down, raising your legs slightly if necessary.
5. Lift your hands about six inches off the mat next to your body, palms down, with your arms and wrists straight, reaching away from your shoulders with your fingertips.

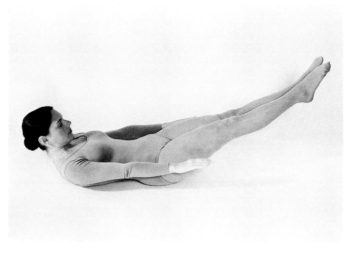

If you do a hundred, you will take ten deep breaths.

Movement

6. Pump your arms up and down rapidly a few inches (toward the ceiling and toward the mat) in short, vigorous motions for five counts.
7. Continue in groups of five for up to one hundred pumps.

Breathing

Breathe IN for five pumping motions.
    OUT for five pumping motions.

Checkpoints

1. Keep yourself firmly anchored to the mat.
2. Navel to spine.
3. Focus on your center. No stomach bulge.
4. Empty your lungs completely with each breath.
5. Don't hunch your shoulders. Reach with your fingertips.
6. As you progress, your legs will be lower, until your toes are on a line with your eyes. But remember to keep your back anchored to the mat.

ROLL-UP

You will need a bar about a yard long. A broomstick will do, or a yardstick, or an umbrella. If you don't have something around, pretend you have a bar in your hands as you do the movement.

Anchoring and Position

1. Lie flat on your back. Legs together, feet flexed.
2. Holding the bar in both hands, put your hands on the mat over your head, arms straight.
3. Spine to mat. Navel to spine.
4. Stretch long and thin from your hands to your heels.

Movement

5. Reaching out of your shoulders as if someone were pulling on the bar, lift your arms from the mat. Lift your head, too, keeping your ears between your arms.
6. Roll up by bringing your head between your upraised arms as if you were looking through a window.
7. Keep your arms moving, imagining someone pulling on the bar, until your hands are aimed at a point just above and beyond your feet. At the same time, continue to roll up, lifting one vertebra at a time off the mat. Let your hands pull you forward until you can go no further. Your chin is on your chest, your heels pushing away from your hips. Navel to spine.
8. Reverse the movement, rolling back down one vertebra at a time. Pinch your buttocks tight and push your heels away from your hips, while visualizing someone holding the bar, lowering you gently to the mat.
9. Keep your chin on your chest and your navel pressed toward your spine.
10. When your shoulderblades reach the mat, start to bring your arms overhead, reaching out, and lower your head, so that you return to Position.

Do up to five Roll-Ups.

Breathing

Breathe IN as you roll up, until you reach a sitting position.

OUT as you reach forward.

IN beginning to roll back.

OUT as you approach the mat.

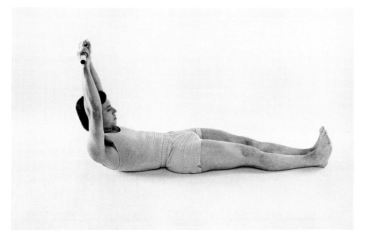

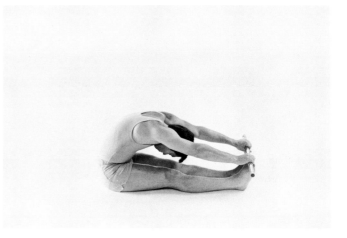

Hints

1. Hook your feet under a piece of furniture to help anchor yourself.
2. Your partner can actually pull on the bar (if you have a partner). Don't pull too hard: pull evenly and gradually. Feel the resistance. Relax.

Checkpoints

1. Keep your stomach *flat*. Center firm. Pay special attention while rolling down.
2. Chin on chest as you roll up and roll down.
3. Push heels away from hips. Feet flexed.
4. One vertebra at a time.

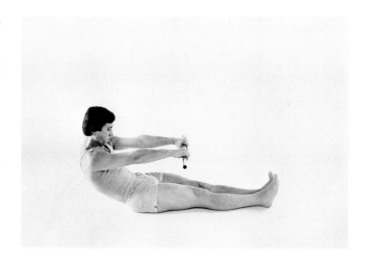

ROLL-OVER

Anchoring

1. Lie on your back with your arms at your sides, palms pressed to the mat.

2. Stretch your neck long and press the base of your skull to the mat.

3. You are anchored from palms to shoulders, along the line across your shoulders, and at the base of your skull.

Movement

4. In one smooth motion, raise your legs off the mat, straight and together, bending only at the hips. Keep going, raising your hips off the mat and bringing them over your body, rolling your spine up and off the mat until your weight is on your shoulders and the back of your head.

5. Stop when your feet are past your head, your toes just touching the mat or as close to it as they'll come. Keep a firm center.

6. Spread your feet, moving them along the mat (or above it) until they are a comfortable distance apart (no more than shoulder width). Your toes should be pointed softly.

7. Legs straight, reaching out of your hips to your toes, roll your spine back down onto the mat one vertebra at a time. Again, use your center to keep your legs as close to your body as possible, until they have to swing up toward the ceiling on the way back to the mat. As your feet approach the mat, bring them smoothly together.

8. Stop when your feet are together about two inches from the mat, or when your legs reach the point where your back begins to arch, if that's sooner.

9. Do three Roll-Overs this way, then do three more with your leg position reversed:

   (a) Bring your legs *up* spread apart.
   (b) When your feet are touching the mat (beyond your head), move your feet together.
   (c) Roll down slowly with your legs together. Concentrate on keeping your knees close to your face on the way down.

Breathing

Breathe IN on the way down.

OUT on the way up.

Checkpoints

1. Navel to spine; stomach flat. Watch for bulge, especially when your legs are more or less pointing at the ceiling.

2. Palms flat.

3. Neck long. Base of skull to mat.

4. Legs straight. Reach out with your toes.

5. Legs close to body on the way down.

6. When your legs are together, hold an imaginary dollar bill between your knees.

7. Don't roll over too far on your neck.

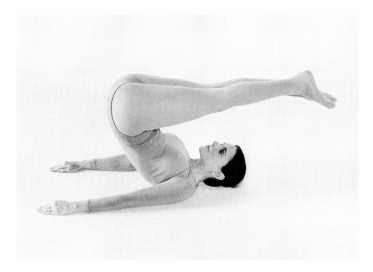 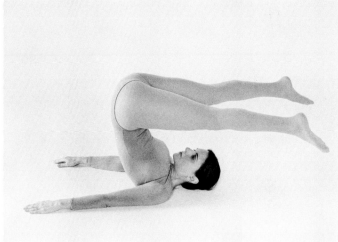

LEG CIRCLES

Anchoring

1. Lie flat on your back, arms by your sides, palms pressed to mat. Legs together.
2. Spine to mat. Navel to spine.
3. Stretch your neck long and press the base of your skull into the mat.
4. Feel yourself anchored along your spine and your arms and hands.

Position

5. Raise your right leg as high as you can, keeping your spine anchored firmly to the mat.
6. Both legs are straight. You can either flex your feet or point them. It is good to alternate from time to time.

Movement

7. Make a circle with your leg—across your body, down toward the mat, out and up.
8. Hold for a moment. Think of stretching your leg toward your face (but don't bend your knee).
9. Do three to five circles, then reverse direction.

Each leg does five circles in each direction.

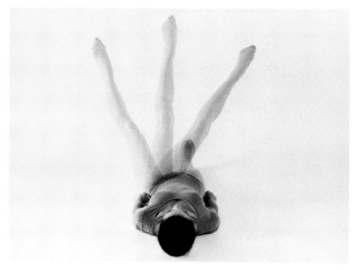

Breathing

Breathe OUT for the first half of the Leg Circle.

IN as you swing your leg back up.

Checkpoints

1. Legs straight (especially the raised one).
2. Spine to mat.
3. Navel to spine. Firm center. No stomach bulge.
4. Don't let your neck arch. Skull to mat and neck long.
5. Use your palms to keep from rocking from side to side (press palms to mat).

ROLLING (LIKE A BALL)

Position

1. Sit on the mat and bring your knees to your chest. (You should be near the end of the mat.)

2. Navel to spine. Round your back and wrap your arms around your legs. Grasp your left ankle with your right hand and your right wrist with your left hand.

3. Bring your heels close to your bottom and lower your chin to your chest. Press your head down between your knees as far as it will go. Tighten your arms around your legs.

Movement

4. Roll all the way back like a ball until you come to rest on your shoulders and neck. Stay tight.

5. Pull down firmly on your legs with your arms to help you start rolling back up without uncurling.

6. Roll all the way back up to Position.

Roll back and forth rhythmically eight to ten times.

Breathing

Breathe IN as you roll backward.

OUT as you roll up.

Checkpoints

1. Navel to spine. Focus on your center.

2. Keep your head down, clamped between your knees.

3. Heels close to bottom.

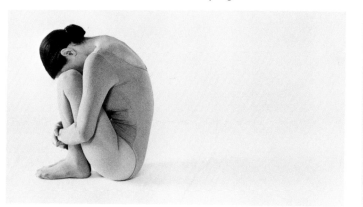 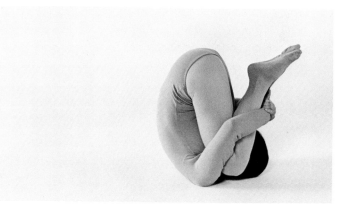

SINGLE-LEG STRETCH

Anchoring

1. Lie flat on your back. Legs straight, toes softly pointed.
2. Navel to spine. Chin on chest.
3. You are anchored where your spine is pressed to the mat.

Position

4. Bring your right knee to your chest; grasp your ankle with your right hand and your knee with your left. Your elbows should be out from your body and raised.
5. Raise your left foot off the mat just high enough to keep your back from arching, stretching out of your hip.

Movement

6. Switch the positions of your legs—reaching long with the toes of your right foot as you bend your left knee close to your chest, grasping your left knee with your right hand and your ankle with your left.
7. Pull the left leg as close to your chest as you can, while reaching as long as possible with your right foot.

Do five to eight stretches with each leg, alternating.

Breathing

Breathe IN for two Leg Stretches.

OUT for two.

Rhythm is essential.

Both inhalation and exhalation are *long* and *gradual*.

Be sure to force all the air from your lungs on the exhalation.

Checkpoints

1. Toes softly pointed.
2. Navel to spine. Firm center.
3. Your shoulders should be relaxed. Don't let them hunch up. Elbows raised.
4. Head forward. Chin on chest.

Ideally, your feet should almost skim the mat, with your foot at eye level when it is fully extended. Try to bring your raised knee to your nose without raising your back from the mat.

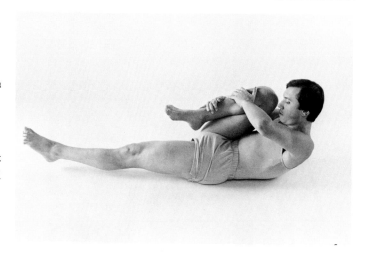

DOUBLE-LEG STRETCH

You can move directly into Position from the Single-Leg Stretch.

Position

1. From the Single-Leg Stretch, smoothly bend your extended leg close to your chest. Grasp your shins and press both legs to your chest, forcing out all the air in your lungs. Focus on your firm center.

Movement

2. Extend *both* legs the way you extended one for the Single-Leg Stretch. Keep your legs together and your feet softly pointed.
3. At the same time, sweep your hands up toward the ceiling and over (behind) your head, keeping them shoulder width or closer, fingers reaching long.
4. Stretch long and thin, from fingertips to toes. Don't let your back arch. Keep your head up, chin on chest.
5. Sweep your arms out to your sides, keeping them close to the mat, while bending your knees to return to Position.

Do up to five smooth, graceful stretches.

Breathing

Breathe IN as you stretch your arms and legs OUT.

OUT as you bring your legs and arms IN toward your chest.

Press your legs to your chest to force all the air from your lungs.

Checkpoints

1. Keep your toes pointed, feet and legs together.
2. Watch your stomach! No bulge. (If you can't see it, sense it. Pay attention to your navel.)
3. Your shoulders should be relaxed. Don't let them hunch up.
4. Keep the movement smooth and flowing.
5. Your arms should stretch long, fingers pointed, making a wide, graceful circle.
6. Keep your head forward (chin on chest) as much as you can.
7. Don't let your back arch.

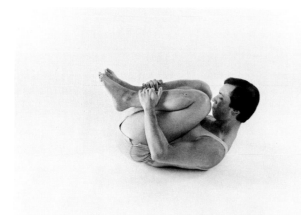

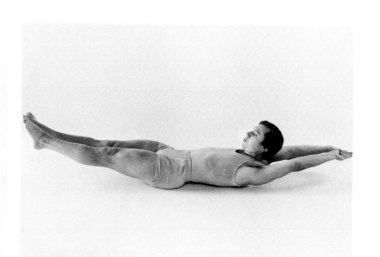

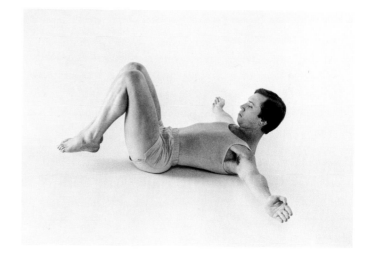

SPINE STRETCH

In spite of its name, this is basically a breathing exercise.

Anchoring and Position

1. Sit on the mat with your legs spread a little more than shoulder width, feet flexed.
2. Anchor your buttocks to the mat. Sit up out of your hips. Navel to spine.

Movement

3. Curl in and down. Aim the top of your head toward your center.
4. At the same time, stretch forward with your hands, reaching past an imaginary line running between your feet.
5. While you are stretching outward and curling in, keep your navel pressed to your spine.

6. When you can go no farther, pause and press your knees toward the mat pushing out through your heels and reaching with your fingers.
7. Force out whatever breath remains in your lungs, reaching farther forward.
8. Return to Position by reversing the motion, concentrating on keeping your head curled down, even as you sit up.

Do up to five stretches, paying particular attention to your breathing.

Breathing

Breathe IN when returning to Position.

OUT on the way down, concentrating on forcing the air from your lungs on the farthest point of your stretch.

Checkpoints

1. Don't hunch your shoulders or let them rise as you reach forward.

2. Navel to spine.

3. Force all the air from your lungs—one, two, three—while reaching and curling.

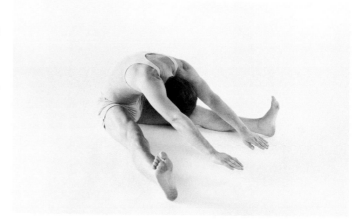

OPEN-LEG ROCKER I

Position

1. Sit on the mat with your knees bent so your feet are to-gether and close to your bottom, with your toes softly pointed and touching the mat.
2. Grasp the tops of your ankles, with your elbows between your knees.
3. Sit tall. Navel to spine.
4. Lift your toes off the mat. Feel yourself balanced on the base of your spine.

Movement

5. Straighten your legs to form a V. Your feet should be about at eye level, not much farther apart than the width of your shoulders.
6. Bring your feet together.
7. Spread your feet to form a V again.
8. Bend your knees and return to Position.

Repeat four times.

Breathing

Breathe IN as you straighten your legs and bring your feet together.

OUT as you form the second V and return to Position.

Hints

1. At first, you may not be able to straighten your legs if you keep your hands on your ankles. If so, grasp your legs higher up (along the shins).
2. If you find it difficult to maintain your balance, practice sitting in Position with your feet off the mat.

Checkpoints

1. Back straight, neck long.
2. Don't slump.
3. Toes pointed.
4. Navel to spine. No stomach bulge.
5. Keep your shoulders relaxed. Don't let them hunch up.

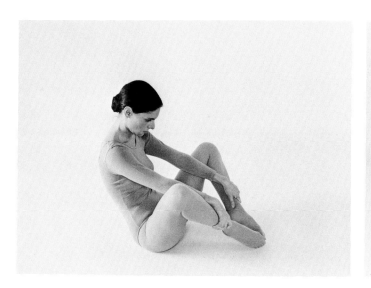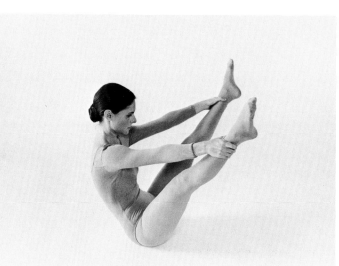

OPEN-LEG ROCKER II

Position

1. Sit on the mat with your knees bent, feet together and close to your bottom, toes softly pointed and touching the mat.

2. Grasp your ankles, elbows between your knees. Sit tall. Navel to spine.

3. Straighten your legs to form a V. Toes still softly pointed, about eye level. Arms straight.

4. Chin on chest.

Movement

5. Under full control, roll backward along your spine, keeping your arms and legs straight.

6. Roll back smoothly until your weight is on your shoulders and your toes are just above the mat. Hold for a second.

7. Roll back up until you are balanced in Position.

Repeat up to five times. Three done perfectly is enough.

Breathing

Breathe IN on the way back.

OUT on the way up.

Hints

1. It's all in your abdomen, especially on the way up. Keep your center as firm as possible, tightening it even more to stop and to give yourself impetus on your way back to Position.

2. If you come up too rapidly, you'll overbalance and fall forward out of control. You can feel this as it starts to happen. Control it by bending your knees, tightening your center, and concentrating on maintaining your balance.

3. This is basically a very graceful exercise. Everything should be done with control. Don't throw yourself around.

Checkpoints

1. Firm center. Chin on chest.
2. Straight legs. Reach out of your hips with your toes.
3. Straight arms.
4. Watch out for wobble! This is an exercise in which your imbalances will make themselves obvious. Do your best to control any tendency to go to one side or the other, especially on the way up.
5. If you can't come up, you've rolled back too far.

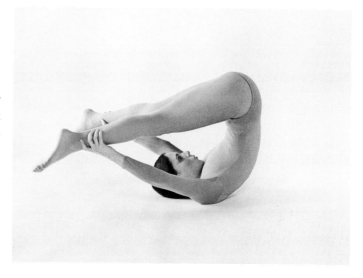

CORKSCREW I

If you have a back problem, proceed with special care.

Anchoring

1. Lie flat on your back with your arms at your sides, your legs straight, and your toes softly pointed. Stretch your neck out of your shoulders.
2. Anchor yourself by pressing your palms and the base of your skull into the mat.

Position

3. Raise your legs to a ninety-degree angle with your body.
4. With your legs straight, reach for the ceiling with your toes. Imagine you are holding a dollar bill between your knees.
5. Spine to mat, navel to spine.

Movement

6. Keeping both hips glued to the mat, make a circle in the air with your feet and legs, starting by swinging them to the left. Keep the dollar bill clamped between your knees.

7. When the first circle is complete do another in the other direction, starting to the right.

Do three to five pairs of circles. As you get better, increase the size of your circles, but keep your hips glued to the mat. When you are comfortable making circles about twice hip width in diameter, move on to Corkscrew II.

Breathing

Breathe IN for one circle.
  OUT for one circle.

Hints

1. If you can't raise your legs straight up, bend your knees to your chest and then push your toes up toward the ceiling.
2. Concentrate on keeping your anchor solid and your center firm at all times.

Checkpoints

1. Legs straight, toes softly pointed.
2. Hold that dollar bill between your knees.
3. Navel to spine. Firm center.
4. Neck long. Base of skull pressed into mat.
5. Don't hunch your shoulders.

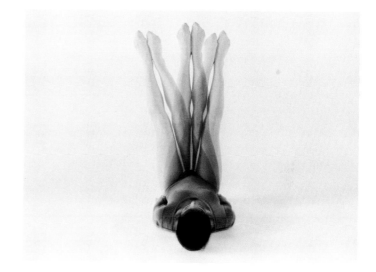

CORKSCREW II

In this version of the Corkscrew, you raise your hip off the mat.

Anchoring

1. Lie flat on your back with your arms at your sides, your legs straight, and your toes softly pointed. Stretch your neck out of your shoulders.

2. Anchor yourself by pressing your palms and the base of your skull into the mat.

Position

3. Raise your legs to a ninety-degree angle with your body.

4. With your legs straight, reach for the ceiling with your toes. Imagine you are holding a dollar bill between your knees.

5. Spine to mat, navel to spine.

Movement

6. Make a circle in the air with your feet and legs, starting by swinging them to the left. Keep the dollar bill clamped between your knees.

7. As you move your legs into a circle to the left, let your right hip come up off the mat slightly. Maintain your anchor by pressing your palms and the back of your skull to the mat. Keep navel to spine and your center very firm.

8. As your legs pass center and swing to the right, your right hip rolls down and your left hip rolls up slightly. Keep your spine on the mat. Your hips are flat when you complete the circle.

9. Reverse.

Do three to five pairs of circles. Increase the size of your circles as you get stronger.

Breathing

Breathe IN for the first half of each circle.

OUT for the second half of the circle.

Hint

Concentrate on keeping your anchor solid and your center firm at all times.

Checkpoints

1. Legs straight, toes softly pointed.
2. Hold that dollar bill between your knees.
3. Navel to spine. Firm center.
4. Neck long. Base of skull pressed into mat.
5. Don't hunch your shoulders.
6. Watch out for stomach bulge when you raise your hip.

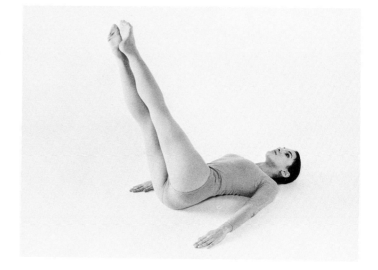

CORKSCREW III

This is the version that gives the exercise its name. It requires a strong back.

Anchoring

1. Lie flat on your back with your arms at your sides, your legs straight, and your toes softly pointed. Stretch your neck out of your shoulders.

2. Anchor yourself by pressing your palms and the base of your skull into the mat.

Position

3. Raise your legs, straight, and together, and keep them moving until your hips come up off the mat and your weight is on your shoulders. Your feet will be near the mat, beyond your head.

4. Adjust your position, pulling your knees close to your face and pressing your vertebrae one at a time back down onto the mat. This will bring your hips toward the mat again (but not all the way), and it will make your feet rise.

5. When you are correctly in position, your weight should be on your back, not your head. Navel to spine. Legs straight and together, toes softly pointed. Knees to nose. You may have to experiment to find the proper balance.

Movement

6. Remaining anchored by your back, palms, and head, twist the part of your body that's off the mat: Your hips move right, your feet (together) left.

7. When you can't twist any more, begin to make a circle with your legs, continuing to move your feet to the left, then down and out toward the mat, around to the right, and up. Twist back into Position.

8. Reverse, moving your feet to the right this time as you twist, circle, untwist.

Do three very controlled Corkscrews.

Breathing

Breathe IN as you Corkscrew out and down.

OUT as your legs come up and back to Position.

Hints

1. The higher your hips are from the mat, the harder it is to do the Corkscrew.

2. Larger circles also make it harder.

3. Your palms are an important brace at either side of your body.

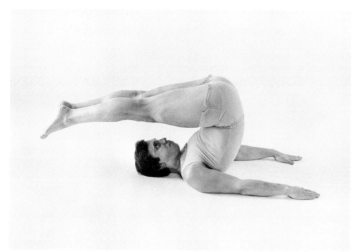

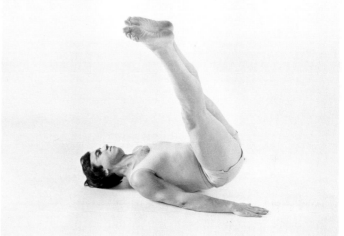

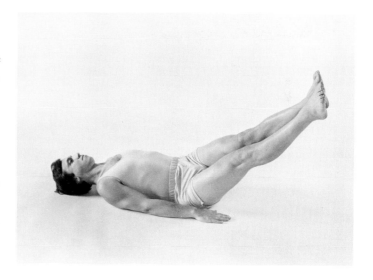

4. Control is vital. If you attempt too much, you'll be flopping all over the mat, and you could hurt your back. Approach this one gradually.

Checkpoints

1. Very firm center.
2. No stomach bulge. Be especially careful as your legs approach the mat and begin to circle up again.
3. Legs straight and together. Hold a dollar bill between your knees.
4. Don't tense your neck; don't hunch your shoulders.

THE SAW

Anchoring

1. Sit on the mat with your legs spread a little more than shoulder width.
2. Legs straight, heels pushed out, feet flexed.
3. You are anchored firmly to the mat from buttocks to heels.

Position

4. Visualize a pole running from the base of your spine up through the top of your head. Slide your head up the pole as far as possible, sitting up out of your hips. Don't arch your back.
5. Raise your arms straight out at your sides, parallel to the floor, palms down, fingertips reaching outward.

Movement

6. Rotate your body, at the same time reaching *past* your left foot with your right hand, so that your pinky and the edge of your hand slide along the base of your little toe, as if you were sawing off your toes with the edge of your hand.

7. As your right hand reaches forward, stretch your left hand out behind you, raising it as high as possible.
8. Let your head follow your forward arm. Keep your buttocks anchored to the mat.
9. Return to Position by reversing the motion of 6–8. Move smoothly and with control, sitting up out of your hips.
10. Reverse, sawing at your right toes with your left hand and stretching up and back with your right.

Repeat three to five times to each side.

Breathing

Start by breathing IN as you push your head up the pole.

Push the air gradually and steadily OUT of your lungs as you reach forward.

Breathe IN while returning to Position.

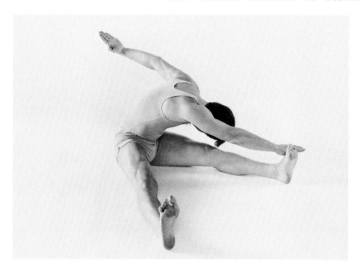

In addition to the Corkscrew, the three exercises that follow, together with their variations, should be approached with special care by people with back problems.

Do not even attempt the Swan Dive I, Swan Dive II, One-Leg Kick, or Double-Leg Kick unless you are sure your back is strong enough.

Checkpoints

1. Legs straight. Push out through your heels.
2. Do not let your hip rise as you reach forward.
3. Each time you return to Position, try to slide your head up that pole, sitting up out of your hips, but not arching your back.
4. Don't hunch your shoulders.
5. Keep your navel glued to your spine.
6. Make sure your reaching hand does not drop below the level of your toes.

SWAN DIVE I

Position

1. Lie flat on your stomach, with your legs stretched straight and your toes softly pointed.

2. Put your palms flat on the mat, directly under your shoulders.

3. Stretch your feet out farther, pushing out from your hips through your toes, lifting your feet slightly off the mat.

4. At the same time, straighten your arms, lifting your torso from the mat. With your head back, lift your chestbone to the ceiling, pinching your buttocks tight to help elevate your torso and your feet. Feel the stretch from the top of your head through your chest and hips and out to your toes.

Movement

5. Bend your arms and let yourself rock forward as if your breastbone were the rim of a wheel. Stay stretched out as in instruction 4; head back, neck long, chest lifted, legs reaching.

6. When you've rocked forward onto your upper chest, push with your hands to help you rock back to Position.

Breathing

Breathe IN on the way up.

OUT on the way down.

Hints

1. Concentrate on getting as much stretch as you can.

2. If you can't straighten your arms at first, work up to it.

Checkpoints

1. Pinch your buttocks tight.

2. Don't let your rib cage and chest sink down.

3. Don't let your shoulders hunch: reach out of your neck.

4. Reach out of your lower back with your legs.

5. Don't collapse on the way down.

Note for Men

This exercise may be more comfortable if you do it with a pad or pillow under your hips.

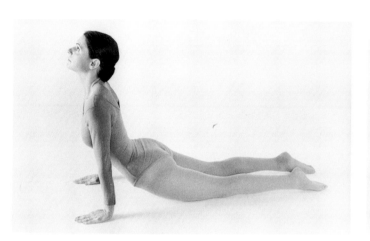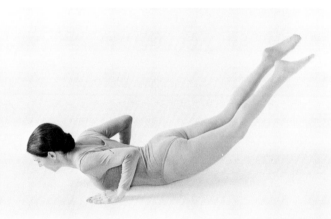

SWAN DIVE II

Position

1. Lie flat on your stomach, with your legs stretched straight and your toes softly pointed.

2. Put your palms flat on the mat, directly under your shoulders.

3. Stretch your feet out farther, pushing out from your hips through your toes, lifting your feet slightly off the mat.

4. At the same time, straighten your arms, lifting your torso from the mat. With your head back, lift your chestbone to the ceiling, pinching your buttocks tight to help elevate your torso and your feet. Feel the stretch from the top of your head through your chest and hips and out to your toes.

Movement

5. Lift your hands clear of the mat and let yourself rock forward as if your breastbone were the rim of a wheel. As you rock forward, extend your arms smoothly in front of you and outward to the sides, palms up. They should feel like wings.

6. When you've rocked forward onto your upper chest, tighten your back, pinch your buttocks harder, reach long through your toes, and lift with head, chest, and arms, so that you rock back as far as possible.

7. Let yourself rock forward again, but hold the shape of your body. Don't relax.

Rock back and forth three to six times.

Breathing

Breathe IN on the way up.
OUT on the way down.

Hints

1. The power for this exercise is focused in your buttocks.

2. Smoothness counts. The idea is to establish a back-and-forth rhythm. If you do it right, you will lift your chest higher each time. It's like pumping a swing (but not as abrupt).

Checkpoints

1. Pinch your buttocks tight.
2. Keep your arms high and straight, arms toward the ceiling.
3. Lift with head and chest.
4. Legs straight, feet together, toes reaching.
5. Smooth! Beware of convulsive or jerky motions trying to propel yourself upward, especially early in your experience with this movement.
6. Chin up. Mouth closed.

Note for Men

This exercise may be more comfortable if you do it with a pad or a pillow under your hips. Center your hipbones on the pad: if it's too far forward, it will interfere with your rocking properly.

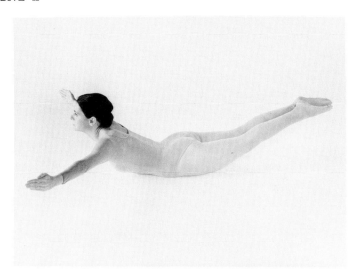

SINGLE-LEG KICK

Anchoring

1. Lie flat on your stomach, with your legs stretched straight and your toes pointed softly.

2. Put your elbows on the mat directly under your shoulders.

3. Clench your fists and place them on the mat straight out ahead of your elbows, like the Sphinx.

4. Your anchor is your fists, forearms, and the line across your hips.

Position

5. Firmly anchored, lift your breastbone as high toward the ceiling as you can, stretching out of your hips.

6. Head back, chin to ceiling. Keeping your mouth closed firms your chin.

7. Push your toes as far from your hips as you can, with your feet slightly off the mat. Pinch your buttocks tight.

Movement

8. Keeping your toes pointed softly, kick your right foot rapidly toward your buttocks, twice. Kick, kick.

9. Then stretch your right leg out and down toward the mat, reaching out of your lower back. Simultaneously, swing your left leg upward, beginning two rapid kicks at your buttocks. Both legs should be in motion at the same time.

Do three to five kick-kicks with each leg.

Alternate legs rapidly and with good rhythm and coordination.

The kicks should be crisp and snappy.

Breathing

Breathe IN on right-leg kicks.

OUT on left-leg kicks.

Checkpoints

1. Pinch your buttocks.
2. Lift your breastbone to the ceiling.
3. Keep your head reaching back. Mouth closed.
4. Try not to sink into your hips.
5. Crisp kicks.
6. Coordinate so that your legs are passing each other when you alternate (i.e., *don't* put the right foot all the way back into Position before you start kicking with your left).
7. Don't let your feet touch the mat.

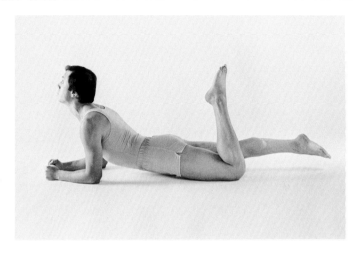

DOUBLE-LEG KICK

Anchoring and Position

1. Lie on your stomach with your right cheek on the mat. legs together, feet softly pointed.

2. Clasp your left hand with your right, behind your back. Place them as high up on your spine as you can.

3. Lower your elbows toward the mat. You may need to move your hands slightly lower on your spine to get your elbows down to the mat. If they still don't touch it, don't strain.

4. Feel yourself anchored to the mat across your hipbones.

Movement

5. Bend both knees and try to kick your buttocks three times with both feet, keeping your knees and feet together. The kicks should be brisk and rapid, without pausing between them.

6. Stretch your clasped hands out behind you, trying to make them reach past your buttocks. At the same time, lift your legs off the mat, stretching out through your toes.

7. Hold for a moment, making yourself long and thin, reaching for the ceiling with your nose, pulling your hands toward your feet.

8. Return to Position with your *left* cheek on the mat this time.

9. Begin kicking again, as in instruction 5. Continue Movement sequence.

Repeat twice to each side. Increase to four times.

Breathing

Breathe OUT as you kick-kick-kick.

IN as you stretch long.

OUT as you return to Position and kick again.

Hints

1. If at the beginning you can't get your elbows down to the mat, concentrate on holding them as low as possible while you kick.

2. As you stretch, pinch your bottom tight to help lift your legs off the mat.

3. Look up at the ceiling to keep your head high.

4. Sense the muscles tightening along your spine when you stretch your hands back.

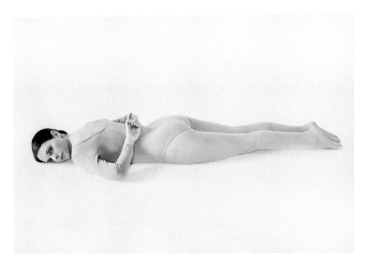

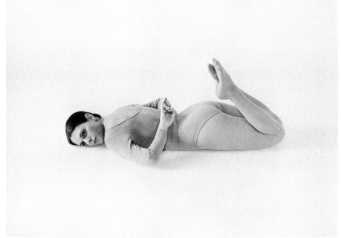

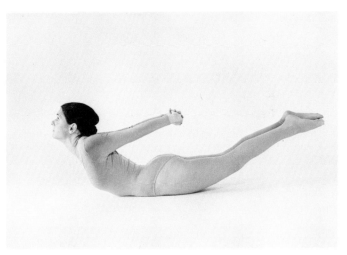

Checkpoints

1. Keep your elbows as low as possible while you are kicking.

2. Kick briskly and with force, but maintain control. Try to make your heels touch your buttocks.

3. Do not interlace your fingers. Simply clasp your left hand with your right (or your right hand with your left, if that is more comfortable).

4. Pinch your bottom.

5. Neck long.

REST POSITION

This is an excellent way to rest and stretch your back after you've done one or more of the preceding three exercises.

Position

1. You are lying on your stomach. Legs together, tops of your feet on the mat. Palms on the mat, arms extended.

Movement

2. Bend your knees and draw your body backward so your bottom is on your heels. Do not raise your head or your hands.

3. As you move, let your back round comfortably. Your arms follow your body, providing a mild stretch for your back and shoulders.

4. Relax.

5. If you want to, bring your hands to your sides and let your knuckles rest easily on the mat.

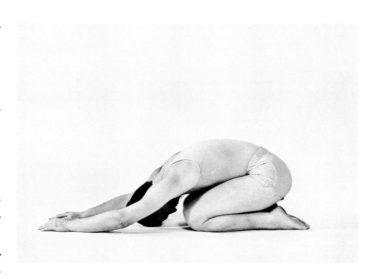

Breathing

Breathe IN and OUT naturally. After a few breaths, concentrate on pushing all the air out of your lungs by prolonging your natural restful exhalation. Don't strain.

Checkpoints

1. Relax.
2. Let your body stretch itself.
3. Watch out for tension in your neck.

NECK PULL

Anchoring and Position

1. Lie flat on your back, hands at the base of your skull, elbows on the mat.
2. Spine to mat, navel to spine.
3. Place your feet hip-width apart on the mat, pushing out with your heels, feet flexed. You are anchored from buttocks to heels.

Movement

4. Roll your head forward until your chin is on your chest.
5. Keep rolling smoothly, bringing your shoulders and back off the mat one vertebra at a time. Think of curling yourself into a tight spiral, keeping your navel glued to your spine. Press your head in toward your navel. Elbows back.
6. When you have rolled up as far as you can, uncurl and sit up straight. Visualize a pole running from the base of your spine through the top of your head: with your elbows high and out at your sides, slide your head as far up the pole as you can. Don't arch your back. Feel your torso lifting out of your hips.
7. Still reaching out of your hips, pinch your buttocks tight and begin to roll down, lowering yourself to the mat one vertebra at a time by reaching out with your chest while pinching your buttocks tighter and keeping your stomach flat. Push your heels away from your hips.
8. Rolling up and rolling down, concentrate on your center. The firmer and stronger it feels, the easier this movement will be.

Do two to five Neck Pulls.

Breathing

Breathe IN as you curl up and then

OUT to get yourself curled as tightly as possible.

IN as you sit up tall. A truly deep breath will help you lift.

OUT on the way down.

Hints

1. At the beginning, it will be helpful if you put your feet under a heavy piece of furniture.
2. Don't strain. Curl up slowly with control.

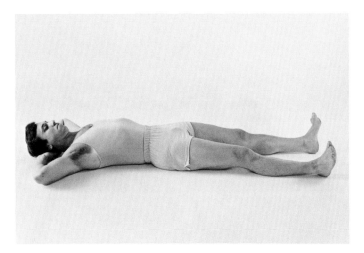
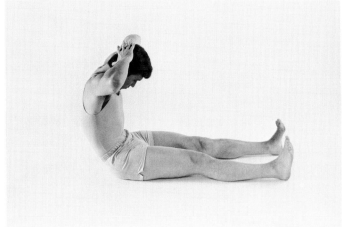

3. If you can't curl up all the way, help yourself into a sitting position and continue the movement: curl yourself down and in, pushing all the air out of your lungs. Sit up tall, reaching out of your hips and taking a deep breath. Begin to curl down. If you feel any strain, relax and lower yourself to the mat.

Checkpoints

1. Don't let your shoulders hunch up.

2. Try to keep your elbows back on a line with your ears.

3. Watch your stomach. The motive power in the Neck Pull comes from tightening your abdominal muscles so

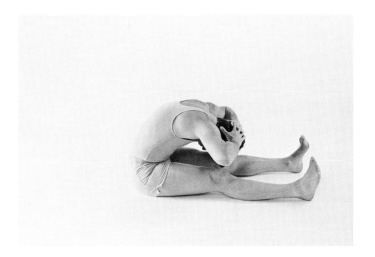

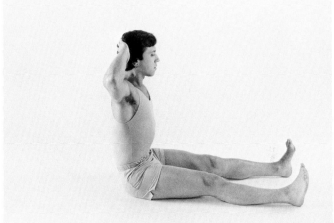

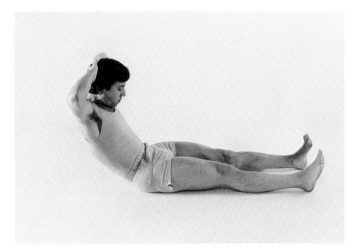

that your stomach is as close to your back as you can make it.

4. Gradually curl up and uncurl. This is *not* a sit-up. Resist the impulse to tighten your abdomen spasmodically.

5. Sit up very tall. Feel the vertical lift in the part of your body between your hipbones and your navel.

SCISSORS

Anchoring and Position

1. Lie flat on your back with arms by your sides. Legs straight and together. Toes softly pointed.

2. Stretch your neck long and press the base of your skull to the mat.

3. Raise your legs to a ninety-degree angle with your body and in the same movement swing your hips up off the mat, reaching for the ceiling with your toes.

4. Put your hands on your back above your hips, elbows on the mat directly below your hands. The higher you can raise your body, the higher you'll be able to place your hands on your back.

5. Your skull, shoulders, and upper arms form a strong base for the Scissors, but the most important support for this movement is your center, not your hands and arms. If you rely on hands and arms, you will not be able to do the movement properly. So:

6. Navel to spine. Pinch your buttocks. Throughout, concentrate especially on maintaining a firm center.

Movement

7. With your toes softly pointed, stretch your toes toward the ceiling.

8. Still stretching upward with your left leg, reach past your bottom with the toes of your right. Straight legs.

9. Let your left leg move slightly in the direction of your head to maintain your balance, but concentrate on moving your right leg as far past your bottom as you can.

10. Reverse, scissoring your legs past each other.

Do three pairs of Scissors.

Breathing

Breathe IN reaching back with the right leg.

OUT reaching back with the left leg.

Checkpoints

1. Navel to spine.

2. Hips motionless. Hold yourself in place with a firm center.

3. Concentrate on stretching your leg past your bottom.

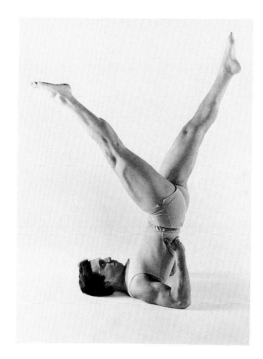

BICYCLE

This has the same name as a familiar exercise, and it looks a little like its namesake, but in fact it is very different. Anchoring and Position are the same as for the Scissors.

Anchoring and Position

1. Lie flat on your back with your arms by your sides. Legs straight and together. Toes softly pointed.

2. Stretch your neck long and press the base of your skull to the mat.

3. Raise your legs to a ninety-degree angle with your body and in the same movement swing your hips up off the mat, reaching for the ceiling with your toes.

4. Put your hands on your back above your hips, elbows on the mat directly below your hands. The higher you can raise your body, the higher you'll be able to place your hands on your back.

5. Your skull, shoulders, and upper arms form a strong base for the Bicycle, but the most important support for this movement is your center, *not* your hands and arms. If you rely on hands and arms, you will not be able to do the movement properly. So:

6. Navel to spine. Pinch your buttocks. Throughout, concentrate especially on maintaining a firm center.

Movement

7. With your toes softly pointed, stretch your toes toward the ceiling.

8. Still reaching upward with your left leg, *bend* your right leg and reach with your toes past your bottom.

9. Keep the right leg moving: your object is to make as big an arc with it as you can, reaching out for the wall and down toward the floor and then straightening the leg to point again at the ceiling.

10. As your right leg moves, stretch tall with your left, which should move slightly toward your head to help you keep balanced.

11. When your right foot is moving up toward the ceiling again, it is time to begin a circle with your left foot. Remember, you are reaching past your bottom for the wall behind you and then for the floor.

Do up to five rotary motions with each foot. Coordinate them so that both feet are moving smoothly at the same time.

NOTE: Your knees should *not* drop toward your face in this exercise. That's how you do the *other* bicycle, which is not part of the Pilates Method.

Breathing

Breathe IN reaching for the floor with your right leg.

OUT reaching for the floor with your left leg.

Hint

The key to keeping your weight off your hands is not just in maintaining a firm center, but in coordinating the movements of your legs so that you are reaching for the ceiling with one foot just as the other sweeps closest to the mat.

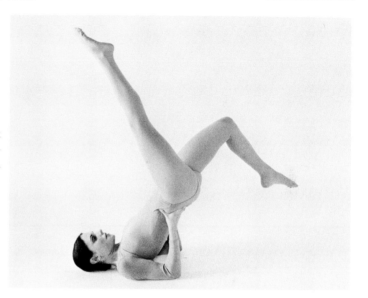

Checkpoints

1. Navel to spine.
2. Back straight and center firm. Hold yourself steady with your abdominal muscles.
3. Reach for the wall and floor with your toes.

SHOULDER BRIDGE

Anchoring and Position

1. Lie on your back, knees bent and feet firmly on the mat.

2. Lift your hips from the mat and support them with a hand under each hipbone. (It may take a little effort; push your hips up with your hands if necessary.) Your elbows should be directly under your hands.

3. Navel to spine. Pinch your buttocks tight.

4. You are anchored from elbows to shoulders, and at the soles of your feet.

Movement

5. Softly point the toe of your right foot and stretch the leg long out of your hip.

6. Kick the leg up smoothly as high as it will go. Leg straight, stretched out of your hip.

7. At the peak of its travel, briskly flex your foot.

8. Lower the leg slowly, pushing constantly outward with your heel, until your foot is just an inch above the mat.

9. Softly point your foot again and repeat. Do three kicks altogether. Return to Position.

10. Do three kicks with your left leg.

Breathing

Breathe IN as your leg kicks up.

OUT, forcing air from your lungs, as you lower your leg.

Checkpoints

1. Keep your pelvis raised high off the mat.

2. Pinch that bottom.

3. Stretch your leg long out of your hip. Toes softly pointed.

4. Skull firmly anchored to the mat.

5. Your hips should be level and motionless. A firm center will help keep them that way.

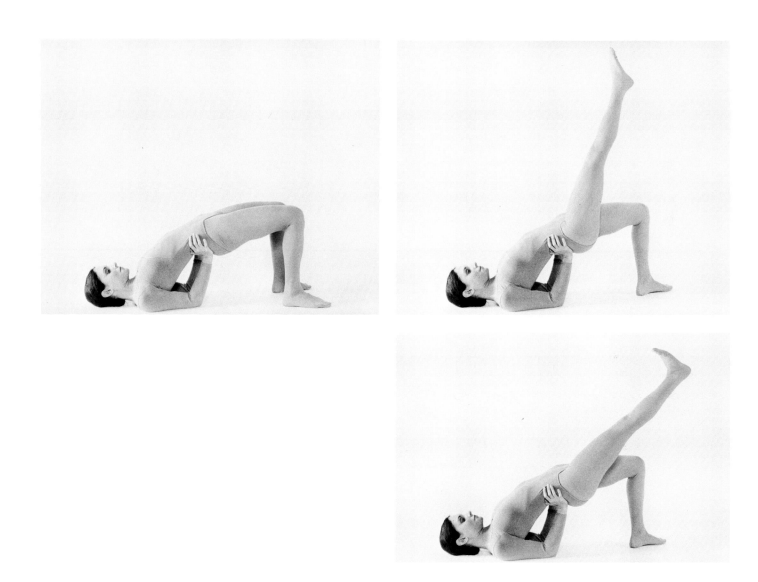

SPINE TWIST

Anchoring

1. Sit straight, with your legs straight and together and your feet flexed.
2. Push your heels as far away from your hips as you can. Feel the stretch. You are anchored from your hips to your heels.

Position

3. Slide your head all the way up the pole that runs from the base of your spine through your spine and neck and out the top of your skull. Feel your torso stretch up out of your hips.
4. Navel to spine.
5. Without letting your shoulders rise, lift your arms straight out at your sides. Imagine another pole through your shoulders and arms: slide your fingertips out along that pole as far from your shoulders as possible.

Movement

6. Turn your head to look at your right wrist and twist your body to the right, leading with your right hand.
7. As you twist, maintain the image of the pole through your arms and shoulders and the one running up your spine. Keep your arms straight and in line with each other and pivot on your spine.

8. When you have twisted as far as you can, give an extra, bouncing twist, then rotate back to Position.
9. Twist the other way.

Do three to five pairs of Twists.

Breathing

Breathe IN as you come to Position.
OUT forcefully when you twist.

Checkpoints

1. The Spine Twist seems so simple that it invites sloppiness. Resist. Do the movement with great precision.
2. Concentrate on lifting your torso out of your hips.
3. Slide your head up that pole.
4. Don't throw your chest forward or arch your spine.
5. Twisting right, don't let your left arm move forward out of line, and watch your right arm when you're twisting left.
6. Twist your head, but don't tilt it.
7. Don't let your shoulders hunch up.
8. Navel to spine.
9. LIFT!

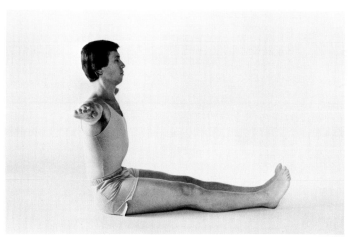 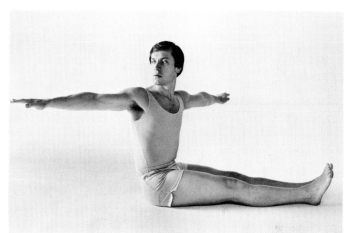

JACKKNIFE

Anchoring

1. Lie flat on your back, hands at your sides, palms pressed flat, neck stretched so the base of your skull is pressed to the mat.

2. Feel anchored at your palms and the base of your skull. Navel to spine.

Position

3. Lift your legs, pressed together, until your toes are pointing straight at the ceiling. Your legs make a right angle with your body.

4. Reach for the ceiling with your toes to straighten your legs; keep your hips on the mat.

Movement

5. Still reaching with your toes, lift your hips and let your straight legs swing very slightly toward your head. Move with control, and stop when your weight is on your shoulderblades and your legs make a forty-five-degree angle with the floor.

6. Lift your toes and hips briskly but smoothly toward the ceiling, pulling your pelvis toward you and pinching your buttocks. Press into the mat with your palms and the back of your head.

7. You will be resting on the nape of your neck. Try to make your body one straight line aiming at the ceiling.

8. Roll your back gradually down onto the mat, one vertebra at a time. Your legs should "jackknife" smoothly through the movement they made on the way up, going to a forty-five-degree angle over your head as they return to Position.

Do three to six Jackknives.

Breathing

Breathe IN on the way up.

OUT on the way down.

Hints

1. To get your legs into Position, first bend your knees to your chest, then straighten your legs.

2. Get your legs as high as you can and your body as straight as it will go by concentrating on pressing your

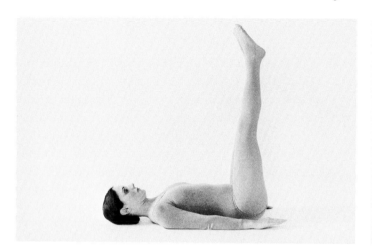

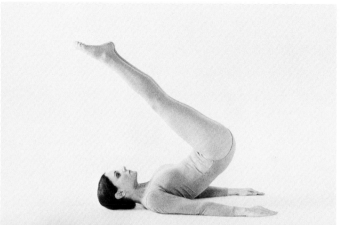

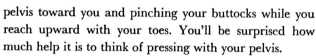

pelvis toward you and pinching your buttocks while you reach upward with your toes. You'll be surprised how much help it is to think of pressing with your pelvis.

3. Concentrate, too, on making your center firmer and tighter. That's where the power is for the Jackknife.

Checkpoints

1. Do the Jacknife as smoothly as possible.
2. Nothing is more important than control; do not jerk yourself off the mat or fall back down.
3. Flat stomach.
4. Don't put too much pressure on your neck.

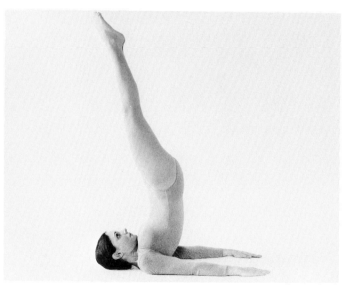

SIDE KICK

Anchoring and Position

1. Lie on your right side with your head resting on your raised right hand, your right elbow extended on a line with your body. You should try to be one straight line, tailbone to elbow.

2. Bend at the hips, so that your legs are still straight, but at an angle with your body, the left leg resting on the right.

3. Brace your left hand on the mat in front of your chest. When you are confident you have mastered the Side Kick in this form, do not place your left hand on the mat. Instead, place it behind your head, with the elbow high and back, maintaining the line of your body.

4. Anchor your entire body to the mat, from foot to elbow.

5. Your left hipbone should be directly above your right, your bottom foot lightly flexed.

6. Navel to spine. Concentrate on maintaining a firm center.

Movement

7. With your left (top) foot softly pointed, stretch the leg, reaching out of your hip. Your foot should be exactly at hip level.

8. Kick your left leg forward, keeping it at hip level off the mat. The kick is in two motions—the first, a long sweeping kick as "high" (toward your face) as you can comfortably go. The second part is a little bounce immediately following the first, pushing the foot a little farther.

9. Sweep your leg back, your foot still lightly pointed, still at hip level, reaching out of your hip, kicking as far backward as you can (past your anchored leg). Again, there is a second, bouncing, extra kick.

10. Immediately start a new kick forward.

Note especially: throughout, keep yourself anchored firmly and *try not to move your torso or hips.*

Do up to five kicks, then turn over and do the same number on the other side.

Breathing

Breathe IN as you kick forward.

OUT as you kick back.

Checkpoints

1. Keep your anchor firm and motionless.

2. Navel to spine. Very firm center.

3. Make sure the top hipbone stays directly over the anchored one.

4. Keep your left elbow up and back, in line with your lower shoulder. Don't let your chest or shoulders sag forward.

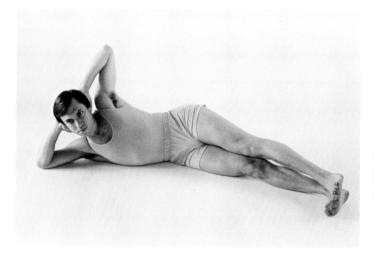

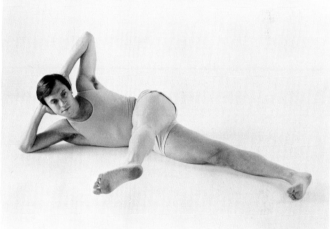

SIDE KICK VARIATION I

Anchoring and Position

1. Remain in Side Kick position. (Review the details, if necessary.)

Movement

2. Bend your top knee and bring your heel toward your buttocks. Reach back to grab your ankle.

3. Holding your heel as close to your buttocks as you can, bring your knee up toward your chest, keeping it at hip level over the mat.

4. As your knee approaches your chest, your foot will come around. Keep pressing your ankle close to your thigh, your thigh close to your chest.

5. When your knee can go no higher, let go of your ankle and grab the underside of your thigh immediately below your knee.

6. Pressing your thigh toward your chest, straighten your leg. (You may have to let your thigh move away from your chest to get your leg straight, but keep up the pressure with your hand.)

7. When your leg is straight, sweep it back over the mat at hip level.

8. When you have kicked as far back as you can without disturbing your solid anchor (one hip directly over the other), again grab your ankle so you can repeat the Movement.

9. Do three kicks and then reverse:

   (a) Sweep your foot forward at hip level.

   (b) Grab the underside of your thigh and press it toward your chest, leg straight.

   (c) Move your hand to your ankle and circle your knee back as far as it will go.

   (d) Let go and kick forward again. Three times altogether.

Turn over and do this variation of the Side Kick three more times, forward and back.

Breathing

Breathe OUT as you bring your knee up and squeeze it to your chest.

IN as you sweep your leg back.

Checkpoints

1. Firm anchor. Don't let your top hip wobble.
2. Navel to spine.
3. Really press your thigh to your chest. Hold it as close to your chest as you can while you straighten your leg.
4. Leg straight, at hip level, as it sweeps over the mat.

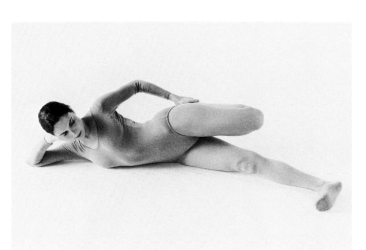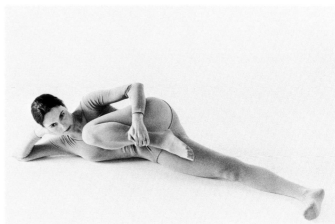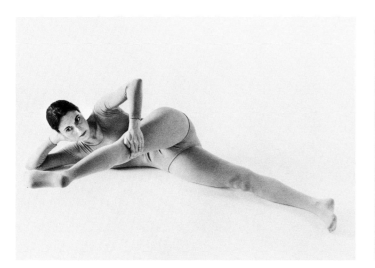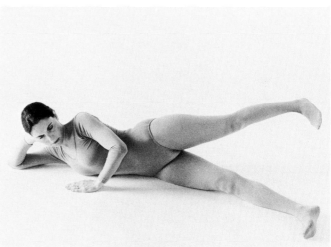

SIDE KICK VARIATION II

Anchoring and Position

1. Remain in Side Kick position. (Review, if necessary.)

Movement

2. Softly point the toes of both feet. Stretch both legs long out of your hips.
3. With your feet together, lift both legs off the mat as high as you can. Make sure your hips stay in line: one directly over the other.
4. Relax.

Lift your legs three times, then turn over and do three on the other side.

Breathing

Breathe IN when you lift your legs.

OUT when you relax.

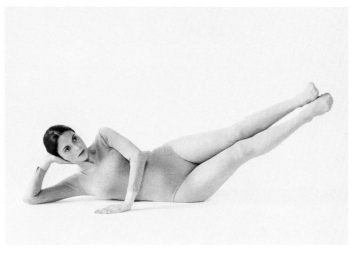

Checkpoints

1. Firm center. Navel to spine.
2. Hips solidly placed. Body steady.
3. Legs straight.
4. Top elbow motionless.

SIDE KICK LIFT

Anchoring and Position

1. Remain in Side Kick position. (Review the details, if necessary.)

Movement

2. Point the toe of your top foot softly and rotate the foot and leg so that the top of your foot is facing the ceiling. *Do not* let your top hip roll backward. This may mean you have to stop rotating your foot when it is only partly facing the ceiling.

3. Stretching out of your hip, kick the leg high, toward the ceiling.

4. At the peak of its travel, flex your foot briskly.

5. Reaching out through your heel, slowly lower your leg to Position.

Do three high kicks and then turn over and do three more on the other side.

Breathing

Breathe IN as you kick up.

OUT slowly and forcefully as you bring your foot down.

NOTE: If you're doing one or more variations of the Side Kick, you can do all of the Movements on one side before you change to the other.

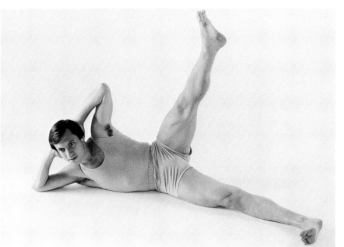
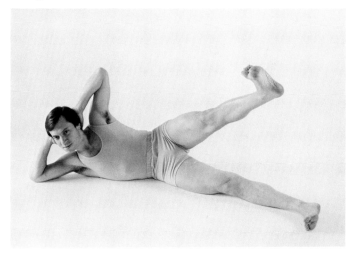

TEASER I

This is a good exercise to do with a partner, at the beginning.

Anchoring and Position

1. Sit on the mat facing a wall or a piece of furniture, or your partner, if you have one.

2. Rest your feet on the wall or the piece of furniture or your partner's thighs (soles flat) so that your legs are at about a forty-five-degree angle with the floor.

3. Lower your torso to the mat so you are lying flat, with your arms at your sides, your palms resting lightly on the mat.

4. Navel to spine.

5. Feel yourself anchored at the lowest point where your hips touch the mat. Your feet are not part of the anchor. They should rest lightly on the wall.

Movement

6. Raise your arms from the mat, the fingertips reaching forward out of your shoulders, pulling you toward your toes.

7. At the same time, keeping your navel pressed to your spine and your body firm and straight, let yourself come up off the mat, so that your body and legs form a V.

8. When you are as close to touching your toes with your fingertips as you can come, pause an instant and then return slowly and with full control to Position.

Start with two or three Teasers and build up to five.

As you get better at it, move away from the wall until your toes barely touch. (Or have your partner hold your toes very lightly.) The purpose of using the wall (or furniture or a partner) is to fix your feet, which should not move at all during the Teaser.

Eventually, you should do the Teaser without the wall completely.

Breathing

Breathe IN on the way up.

OUT on the way down.

Checkpoints

1. Feet motionless.

2. Firm center. Straight body.

3. Reach with your fingertips.

4. Don't let your shoulders rise or hunch up.

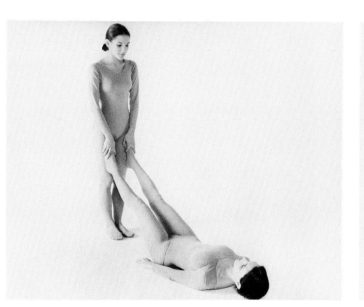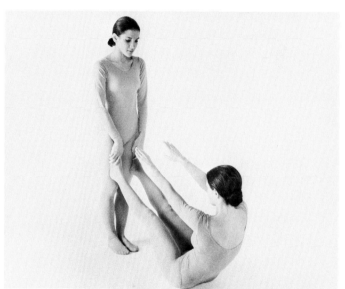

TEASER II

This is the second part of the Teaser. When you're good at Teaser I, add this movement, so you're doing Teaser I and then Teaser II.

Anchoring

1. Sit up tall on the mat with your legs straight and together and your toes softly pointed.
2. Feel yourself anchored at the base of your spine.

Position

3. Press your navel to your spine and make the center of your body as firm as possible.
4. With your back straight, raise your arms at shoulder width and reach forward with your fingertips.
5. Lower your torso backward so your straight back forms about a forty-five-degree angle with the mat.

Movement

6. Keeping your fingertips motionless in the air raise your toes off the mat to touch your fingers (or come as close as you can).
7. Return to Position.

Repeat three to five times.

Breathing

Breathe IN as you bring your toes up.
OUT as you lower them.

Hints

1. No need to hurry.
2. Only do Teaser II after you have become comfortable with Teaser I.

Checkpoints

1. Control. No jerky movements.
2. Stomach flat, firm center.
3. Your shoulders will tend to rise. Don't let them.
4. Straight legs.
5. Toes pointed.
6. Legs together.
7. The Teaser can be a good indicator of unevenness. Pay special attention to keeping your hands and feet exactly even.

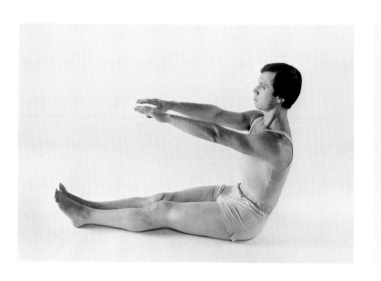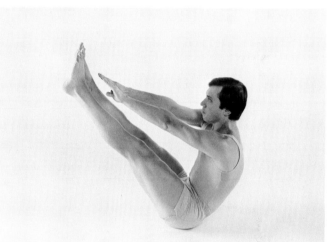

TEASER III

Position

1. Lie flat on your back, legs straight and together, feet softly pointed. Your hands are on the mat over your head, your arms shoulder-width apart.
2. Reach out with your fingertips, stretching long out of your shoulders.

Movements

3. Breaking only at the hips, swing your legs up from the mat. Simultaneously swing up your arms and torso, all in one unit.
4. Reach for your toes with your fingertips.
5. You should try to form a triangle whose three sides are: legs, arms, torso. You are balancing on the mat at the base of your spine. Your legs, arms, and back are straight.
6. Reverse the motion, unfolding smoothly until you are stretched straight out on the mat again. Your legs and your upper body should touch the mat at the same time.

7. Optional: before unfolding, reach up with your arms until your elbows are next to your ears. Now unfold smoothly and with control.

Do up to five Teasers.

Breathing

Breathe IN on the way up.

OUT on the way down.

Checkpoints

1. Navel to spine.
2. Legs straight. Reach out with your toes.
3. Hands even; feet even.

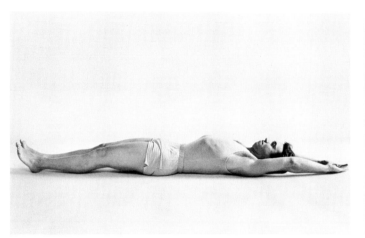

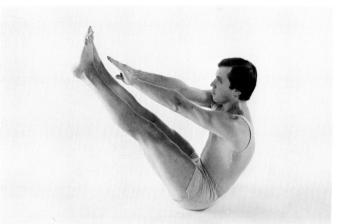

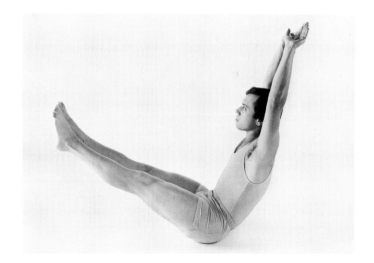

HIP CIRCLES

Anchoring

1. Sit with your arms behind you, palms on the mat.

2. Lean back, spreading your hands and letting them move backward so that they bear a large part of your weight.

3. Keep your arms straight. Your body should be at about a forty-five-degree angle to the mat.

4. Navel to spine. Your anchor is your palms and the base of your spine, connected by a firm center.

Position

5. Bend your knees to your chest

6. Straighten your legs toward the ceiling, keeping knees and feet together, toes softly pointed. Try to keep your knees as close to your nose as possible.

7. Try not to sink into your shoulders or let your chest sink.

Movement

8. Swing your legs in a circle, down to the right, around with your feet near the mat, and up to the left, keeping them together, toes softly pointed.

9. Hold for a moment with your toes reaching for the ceiling and your knees in front of your nose.

10. Reverse, starting to the left and down. Again, hold for a moment in Position.

Do up to five Hip Circles. (Three is plenty to start with.)

Breathing

Breathe IN as you swing your legs down.
OUT as you swing them up.

Hint

1. Make your Hip Circles only as big as you can control them. If your back is arching or you are being pulled out of your anchored position, you're swinging your legs too far. As your center becomes firmer, you can swing your legs farther to each side and closer to the mat.

Checkpoints

1. Navel to spine.
2. Arms straight.
3. Legs together, knees straight, toes softly pointed.
4. You should be motionless above the hips.
5. Watch your stomach: no bulge.
6. Neck long. Don't sink into your shoulders.

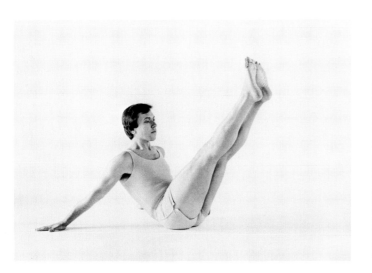

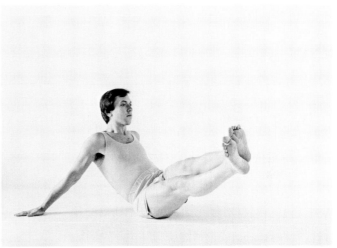

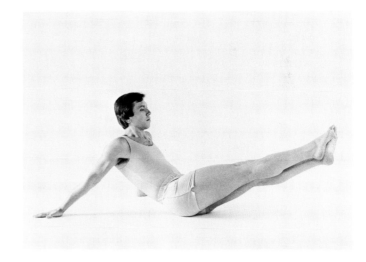

LEG-PULL FRONT

This is an especially good stretch for joggers and runners.

Position

1. Lie flat on your stomach with your legs together, toes on the mat, palms on the mat directly under your shoulders.
2. Navel to spine. Make your center as firm as possible and then straighten your arms so you are in a "push-up" position.
3. Make yourself long and thin and straight—legs, hips, back, neck, and head in a straight line. Pinch your buttocks and make sure your navel is pressed toward your spine and your center is very firm.

Movement

4. Push back into your left heel as if you wanted to make it touch the mat and at the same time lift your right leg. Keep the leg straight and don't break the line of your body. Hips level.
5. Lower your leg, still pushing into your left until you return to Position.

Do four Leg-Pulls on each side.

NOTE: Your body will have a tendency to break at the hips. Keep your center very firm, your hips and torso locked into a straight line.

Breathing

Breathe IN as you raise your leg.

OUT as you lower it.

Checkpoints

1. Center firm.
2. Buttocks pinched.
3. Head, neck, spine, hips, legs all in a line.
4. Stretch your neck out long. Don't hunch your shoulders.
5. Keep the raised leg straight.
6. Keep your pelvis level when you raise your leg.
7. Push hard into your heel. Feel the stretch in the back of your leg.
8. Arms straight.
9. Don't let your hips sink.

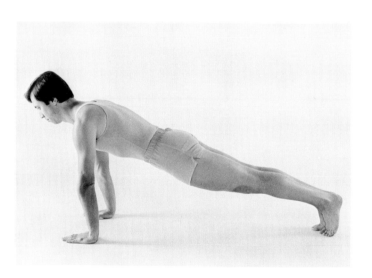 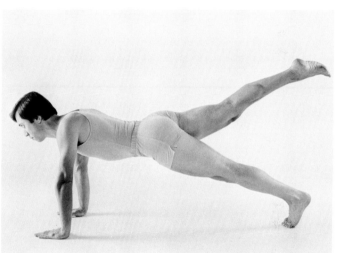

LEG-PULL

Anchoring and Position

1. Sit on the mat, hands by your sides, palms down. Legs straight and together.

2. Raise your hips from the mat, firming your center and pinching your buttocks, so you are supported on your palms and heels. Reach for the mat with your toes.

3. Your arms should be straight and shoulder-width apart, your body stretched into a single straight line from shoulders to toes. Feel solidly anchored.

4. Chin on chest. Navel to spine. Focus on your center.

Movement

5. Without moving your body, kick your right leg as high as you can. Toes softly pointed, leg straight. Reach out of your hip.

6. At the peak of its travel, briskly flex your foot. Lower your leg slowly, pushing out through your heel. Keep your center firm and your hips lifted, so your body remains in a straight line.

7. When your foot is almost at the mat, point the toes and kick up again.

Do three kicks. Repeat with the other leg.

Breathing

Breathe IN kicking your leg up.

OUT lowering it toward the mat.

Hints

1. At first, you may want to let your foot come to rest on the mat between kicks. Keep the leg straight, toes softly pointed.

2. Visualize a sharp hatpin under your bottom. Don't let yourself sink down onto it.

Checkpoints

1. Keep your center firm and your body in a straight line.

2. Legs straight.

3. Chin on chest. Don't let your head sink into your shoulders.

4. Arms straight.

5. Don't let your stomach bulge, especially when you kick up.

6. Keep your bottom off that hatpin.

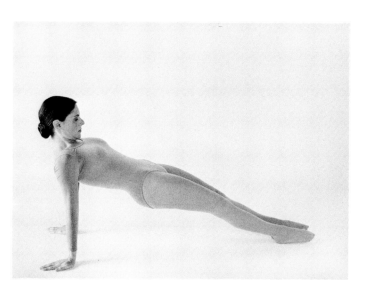

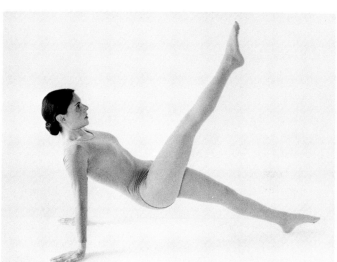

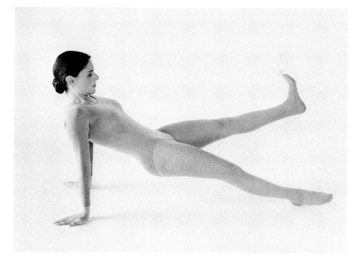

TWIST I

Anchoring and Position

1. Sit sideways with your right palm pressed to the mat next to your right hip, fingers pointing across the mat. Your knees should be bent so that your heels are not far from your left hip. You will be leaning slightly to your right.
2. Navel to spine. Firm center.
3. Twist your left foot so that it is pointing across the mat, with the sole flat on the mat or nearly so, close to your buttocks.
4. Put your right foot behind your left, crossing your feet. The instep of your right foot should rest above your left heel.
5. Your anchor is your right palm and the sole of your left foot.

Movement

6. Swing your bottom smoothly off the mat, around and up until your hip points at the ceiling and your legs are straight. The power for this motion comes from your center.
7. As you swing your hip up, swing your left arm upward, reaching long over your shoulder, the hand moving in a graceful arc, until your upper arm is next to your ear. (Both head and hand end up pointing at the mat.)

8. With complete control reverse the motion and return to Position, concentrating on the long, high sweep of your arm as your hand arcs up toward the ceiling and then down again toward your feet.

Do three smooth, flowing Twists and then change sides so that you are anchored by your left palm and right foot. Do three more.

Breathing

Breathe IN on the way up.
OUT on the way down.

Checkpoints

1. The essence of this exercise is graceful movement. Even though your legs are twisted, your body moves in a smooth arc, like your arm.
2. Your arm reaches long, but it is not rigid. The elbow may bend slightly when your arm is next to your ear.
3. Concentrate on your center, too. Flat and firm. At the peak of the movement, feel your navel being pulled toward the ceiling.

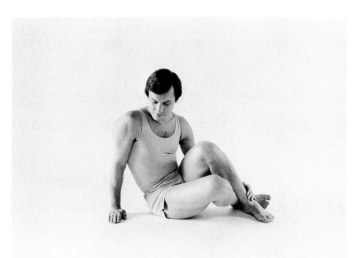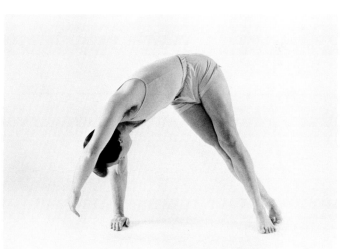

TWIST II

This is a separate exercise, not a substitute for Twist I.

Anchoring and Position

1. Lie on your right side on the mat, legs straight and together, one on top of the other.
2. Raise your torso and prop yourself on your right palm, with your arm straight.
3. Put your left sole as nearly flat on the mat as you can, trying not to move it in toward your body.
4. Put your right foot behind your left, placing your right instep just over your left heel.
5. Your left hand should rest naturally on the mat.
6. Navel to spine. Firm center. Feel yourself anchored by your palm and your left foot.

Movement

7. Lift your left hip straight up toward the ceiling. At the same time, sweep your left hand upward, reaching long toward the ceiling, keeping your hand moving gracefully until your upper arm is next to your ear.
8. As much as possible given the twist in your legs, you should be one long graceful line from your toes to the fingertips of your left hand.

9. Maintaining your firm center and continuing to reach with your left hand, twist your body over with full control so that you are facing the mat. Don't break at the hips.

NOTE: This takes considerable balance and a firm, strong center. Don't twist over any farther than you can without losing your balance. (Reaching out of your shoulder, arm close to your ear, will help you maintain balance.)

10. Twist back, this time trying to face the ceiling.
11. Return to your long, graceful line (instruction 8) and then reverse the motion of instruction 7. Sweep your hand up to the ceiling and then back to the mat in a long, smooth circle, as you lower your hip to the mat.

Do two or three graceful Twists on each side.

Breathing

Breathe IN on the way up.
　　　　OUT as you twist toward the mat.
　　　　IN as you twist toward the ceiling.
　　　　OUT on the way down.

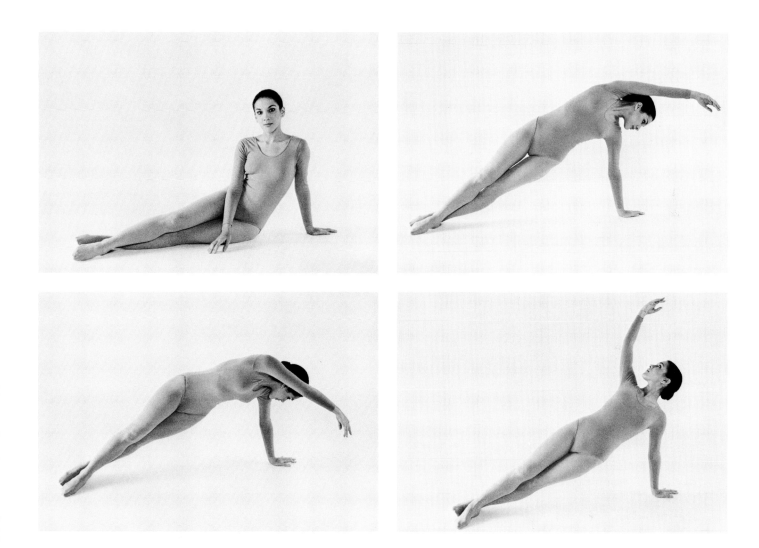

Checkpoints

1. Firm center.

2. Keep your hip lifted toward the ceiling. Don't break in the middle.

3. The essence of this Twist is flowing movement, especially in the smooth, elegant sweep of your arm.

4. Balance. Control.

5. Don't let your head loll. Feel your neck as a long, graceful extension of your spine.

SWIMMING

Anchoring

1. Lie on your stomach with your arms straight in front of you, palms on the mat.
2. Stretch long and thin, from your toes to your fingertips.
3. Anchor your pelvis to the mat.

Position

4. Lift your chest, arms, and legs off the mat, still stretching. Pinch your buttocks.
5. Lift your head high. Look at the ceiling.
6. Lift your right arm and your left leg higher than the other arm and leg.

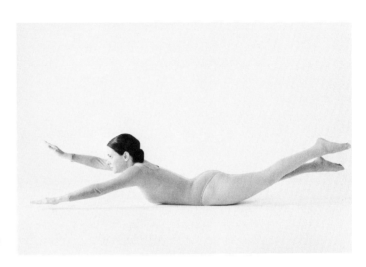

Movement

7. With rapid, brisk motions, alternate lifting your arms and legs. Move arms and legs at the same speed, and keep stretching, so that your knees and elbows do not bend.

Do up to twenty strokes.

Breathing

Breathe IN for five counts.
OUT for five counts.

Checkpoints

1. Arms and legs straight.
2. Stretch long.
3. Pinch your bottom.
4. Long neck: don't hunch your shoulders or let your head sink.
5. Breathe deeply.

BOOMERANG

Position

1. Sit on the mat, hands at your sides, palms on the mat next to your hips, legs straight, toes softly pointed.
2. Keeping your legs straight, cross your right leg over your left at the ankle.
3. Chin on chest. Navel to spine. Sit up out of your hips.

Movement

4. Roll back; use your hands on the mat to help propel you. You should end up with your arms and palms on the mat, resting on your shoulders and neck and the base of your skull. Your crossed legs will be straight out over your face, and your feet will not quite be touching the mat.
5. With a brisk motion uncross and recross your legs, so that your left leg is now over your right.
6. Keep your legs straight, navel to spine, firm center. Lift your arms and roll forward.
7. As you roll, your arms move out to your sides and around behind you. Clasp your hands (if you can) and stretch your arms as far out and up as they will go.
8. Stop your forward motion when your feet are about six inches to a foot above the mat. Balance there for a moment, legs straight, arms stretched out behind you, torso straight.

NOTE: This may take practice. It requires good balance, but it's not as hard as it sounds. The key is your center. It is your abdominal muscles that will stop your forward motion and that will hold you in a balanced position.

9. Complete your roll forward, pressing your torso down onto your legs and raising your arms as high behind you as they will go. Try to touch your head to your legs. Remember to keep navel to spine. Don't let your center collapse.
10. Repeat, recrossing your legs again when you are rolled all the way onto your shoulders.

Do up to five Boomerangs.

Breathing

Breathe IN as you begin to roll back.

OUT when you're reaching the end of your roll and recrossing your legs.

IN rolling up to the point of balance.

OUT as you press your torso over.

Checkpoints

1. Firm center at all times. Navel to spine.
2. Chin on chest.
3. Straight legs.

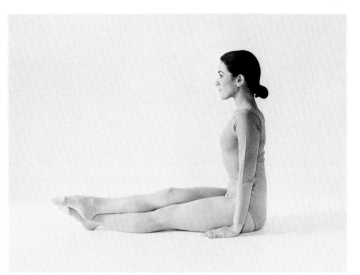
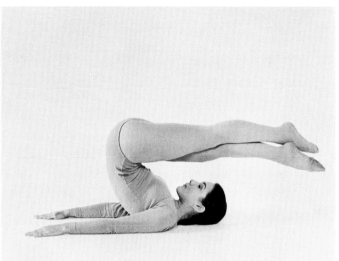
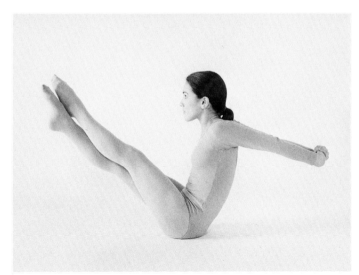
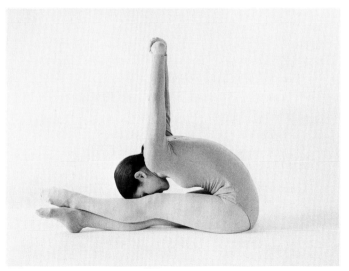

SEAL II

Position

1. Sit with your feet on the mat, your soles pressed together.
2. Bring your arms to your center and reach through the space between your knees, bringing your hands outside your ankles and wrapping them around your feet.
3. Navel to spine. Chin on chest.
4. Lift your toes from the mat so that you are balanced gracefully on the base of your spine.

Movement

5. Roll smoothly onto your back; keep rolling until your weight is on your shoulders and neck, and your toes are an inch from the mat.
6. Balancing where you are, spread your feet apart and then bring them together again. Do this three times. Think of a seal clapping for fish.

7. Roll smoothly back up into Position, with your toes poised over the mat.

Rock back and forth five times.

Breathing

Breathe IN on the way up.
OUT on the way back.

Checkpoints

1. Navel to spine. Firm center.
2. Chin on chest.
3. Smooth motion back and forth.
4. Roll on a straight line. Work to counteract imbalances.

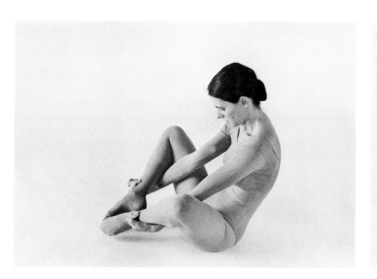 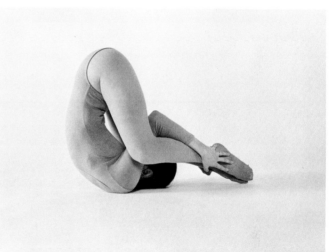

ROCKING

This is an exercise that you need to get the feel of. It is in large part a matter of rhythm and coordination. Don't be discouraged if it takes a while to get the hang of it. WARNING: Proceed carefully. Don't do this unless you have a strong back.

Position

1. Lie on your stomach.
2. Bend your knees and bring your heels as close to your bottom as you can.
3. Reach behind you and grasp your feet with your hands. Your hands should come around the outside of your feet to hold your insteps.

NOTE: You may have difficulty grabbing your feet. It is easier if you do it one foot at a time, leaning to the left as you grab your left foot, to the right as you reach for your right foot.

4. Reach for your toes with the top of your head.

Movement

5. Use the muscles in your legs and back to pull your feet toward the mat. It will help if you relax the muscles across your chest, so that your back curves and you feel your chest open out. Keep pulling with your feet, using your arms to help, so that your chest lifts off the mat.

6. Relax and pull your feet sharply toward your buttocks, rolling forward onto your chest. Keep your mouth closed.

7. At the end of your roll forward, lift your head, pulling your feet toward the mat, so that you begin to rock back again.

Rock back and forth up to five times.

Breathing

Breathe OUT on the way forward.

IN sharply as part of the lifting and pulling that gives you rearward momentum.

Checkpoints

1. Head back.
2. Chest lifted and open.
3. Don't collapse. Think of your body from your collarbone to your knees as being the rim of a wheel.
4. Coordination is important. Develop a rhythm in the movement.
5. While rolling forward, keep your chin clear of the floor.

Note for Men

Use a pillow under your hips.

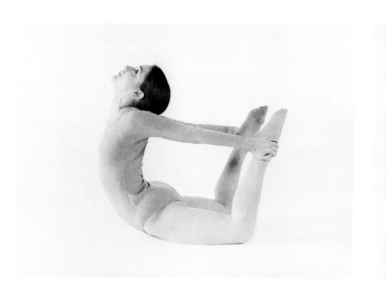 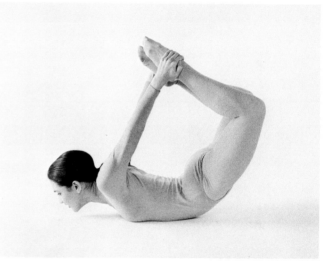

CONTROL BALANCE

Position

1. Lie on your back, arms at shoulder width next to your head, knuckles on the mat. Legs straight and together.

2. Keeping your legs straight, swing them up off the mat and over your head. Keep going until your toes are touching the mat beyond your head (or until they are as close to the mat as you can get them).

3. Grasp your right ankle with both hands.

4. Navel to spine. Firm center.

5. Reach upward with your left leg, stretching out of your hip, while holding your right ankle and keeping your right foot on or near the mat.

Movement

6. Let go of your ankle. Smoothly and with full control reverse the positions of your legs, grasping your left ankle when it approaches the mat. Reach for the ceiling with the toes of your right foot.

7. Lift your pelvis toward the ceiling. Make sure your left leg is straight, the toes softly pointed.

8. Reverse again.

Reach for the ceiling three times with each leg.

Breathing

Breathe IN as one leg reaches up.

OUT as you bring it down and the other one reaches up.

Checkpoints

1. Straight legs.
2. Straight arms.
3. Navel to spine; firm center.
4. Breathe naturally.
5. For an extra stretch, press your toes into the mat. As your raised foot reaches for the ceiling, reach for the mat with the other heel.

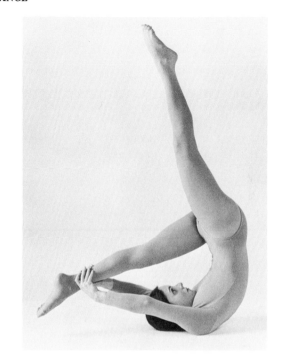

PUSH-UP

Not exactly the one you know.

Position

1. Stand at one end of the mat, with the mat in front of you. Feet hip width. Firm center.
2. Put your hands on the front of your thighs.

Movement

3. Pulling your navel toward your spine, slide your hands down your thighs to your ankles. Bring your head down naturally with the movement so that it is between your arms. Relax your neck and shoulders. Legs straight.
4. Place your hands on the mat and begin to walk them forward, keeping your head between your arms. Legs straight. Navel to spine. Firm center. Keep your heels on the mat as long as possible.
5. As your body straightens, lift your head so that your neck and spine form a straight line. Legs straight. Buttocks pinched. Don't let your body sag.
6. Bend your arms, elbows close to your sides.
7. Touch your chest to the mat and then push yourself up again. Your body should be as straight and firm as an iron bar.
8. Reverse. Walk back with your hands, breaking the line of your body only at the hips. Visualize a string tied to your navel, pulling you up toward the ceiling.
9. When your hands are as close to your feet as you can get them, put them on your legs. Straighten up, walking your hands up your legs as you go.
10. Optional: stretch up as straight and tall as you can, rising onto your toes and reaching for the ceiling with your fingertips.

Breathing

Breathe IN as you walk your hands down your legs.

OUT as you walk your hands along the mat.

IN on the Push-Up downstroke.

OUT on the way up.

IN walking back toward your feet.

OUT on the way up your legs.

Checkpoints

1. Navel to spine at all times.
2. Everything straight as an arrow.
3. Move your head naturally.
4. Don't hunch your shoulders.
5. Elbows close to sides (Movement 6 and 7).

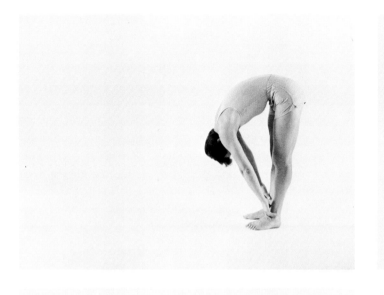
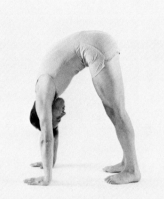
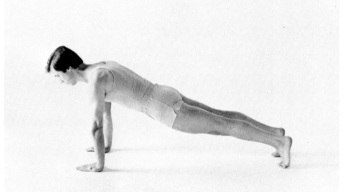
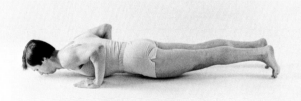

I Don't Feel Like It

Some days, you won't even want to think about exercising. On days like that, unless your reluctance has a physical basis —illness or injury—try to get yourself to do at least a few minutes of Pilates Method movements. You'll be surprised at the results.

Joe put it this way: "Often, you may say to yourself, 'Just this night off.' Suppose the stokers in a steamship took a night off. They might 'get by' with ashes piled high in the furnaces and the machinery beginning to creak and groan. Another 'night off' and the machinery would freeze and the fires die in the furnaces. Remember what the philosopher Schopenhauer said, *'To neglect one's body for any other advantage in life is the greatest of follies.'* Say to yourself, 'I will work ten minutes.' Amazingly enough, once you have started the ten minutes will stretch to more. . . . Your brain clears and your will power works!"

Pressed for Time?

Some of the regulars at the Pilates Studio can do the full program of mat exercises in as little as fifteen minutes, moving briskly but without hurrying. There are even those who say that ten minutes should be enough if you really put your mind to it.

We do not recommend that kind of speed, at least not until you are thoroughly familiar with the method.

You will find that your own program takes a more-or-less constant amount of time if you add new movements as you get better at the ones you already know. From many points of view, at least a half hour per session is a good amount of time to allow yourself.

Some days, you will not have a half hour. Or you will want to do an abbreviated session to refresh yourself. In either case, you have two basic alternatives: (a) you can do the ten exercises of Level 1, or (b) you can select a group of movements from your current program. One caution: If you choose method (b) frequently, try to vary the group of exercises you choose. Getting into a rut, especially when you're in a hurry, is an invitation to sloppiness.

Work the Whole Body

When you select a subgroup of exercises, bear in mind the effect Joe Pilates was trying to achieve in the way he structured the whole program. His idea was to compile a sequence of movements which would work the whole body, calling virtually all of its muscles into play not just once but in a variety of ways, alternately stretching and contracting each muscle group.

To follow that principle, any group of Pilates exercises you pick should have variety and alternation. If you were just doing three exercises, Roll-Up, Neck Pull, and Teaser would be a poor choice. On the other hand, a series like The Hundred, Neck Pull, and Swimming; or Roll-Up, Swan Dive, and Control Balance will refresh you and help maintain your progress, stimulating and stretching your whole body.

Speed and Endurance

To some degree, developing endurance is distinct from developing strength, tone, and suppleness. The added element in endurance training is time.

If you are particularly concerned about developing endurance, there are two ways to enhance the effects of the Pilates Method:

(1) Do a longer session.
(2) Do the same program in a shorter time.

Don't speed up until you're sure you can do it without sacrificing control and precision. Then begin to cut down on the time you take to complete your program of exercises. Always keep in mind the conflict between speed and proper movement.

Although speed can be a problem, there is no virtue in going too slowly. On the contrary: if you go too slowly, you are likely to tense up more than you should as you do the movements. As with how far to go in each movement, you are the best judge of your own body. On the whole, you should maintain a comfortable pace, without any sensation of hurrying or of holding back.

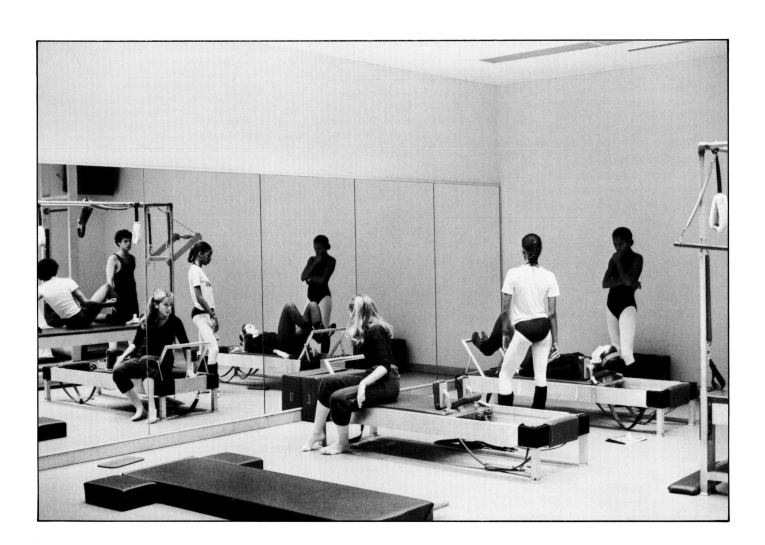

CHAPTER EIGHT

Beyond the Mat Work

Pilates Universal Reformer

When Joe Pilates began to devise his method of conditioning, he was interested in movements that could be done unassisted, without apparatus. It was from his early work that he developed the exercises which were refined and amplified into the program described in chapters Six and Seven.

After Joe was well established in New York, he discovered that some of his students wanted (and could profit from) exercises with a mechanical component. He turned his mind to springs and moving platforms to provide varying amounts of resistance and motion, inventing a variety of devices that could be used for exercises adapted from the mat work.

He built the apparatus, improved them, and patented them. The first and most important, still used in the studio today, he called the Pilates Universal Reformer. Basically, it is a wheeled exercise mat on tracks; the mat's motion is regulated by balancing the pull of springs with the pull exerted on leather straps by the exerciser.

Inevitably, the Universal Reformer—designed to accommodate the mat-work exercises—provided Joe with inspiration for new movements which were not part of the original mat sequence. For this book, we have adapted some of these for you to do at home. Most can be done on the mat; two are standing exercises and require you to use a chair or stool as part of the movement.

Anchoring

1. Lie on your back. Arms at your sides. Legs straight and feet together, toes softly pointed.
2. Navel to spine.
3. Feel your firm center anchored to the mat.

Position

4. Bend your knees and bring your thighs close to your chest.
5. Chin on chest.
6. Bring your knuckles up under your chin. Your elbows should be straight out at your sides.

Movement

7. Simultaneously stretch your arms and legs straight up, reaching for the ceiling with your fingers and your toes, keeping them all roughly parallel.

Instructions 8 and 9 are part of a single, smoothly flowing motion:

8. Sweep your arms and legs out to the side and down, keeping your arms on a line with your shoulders.
9. Bring your legs together and your hands just over your thighs, stretching your fingers and toes long. Your chin is still on your chest. You are focused on your center. Hold for a moment.
10. Return to Position.

Do three complete Backstrokes.

Breathing

Breathe IN as you extend your limbs upward.
    OUT as you sweep them around and down.
    IN again as you bring your legs together and your arms to your sides.
    HOLD for a moment.
    OUT as you return to Position.

Checkpoints

1. Navel to spine at all times. Flat stomach; firm center.
2. Chin on chest.
3. Straight arms and legs. Stretch out of your hips and shoulders.
4. Smooth, flowing motion. Don't hurry.
5. Coordinate breathing carefully, especially the out-in breath that accompanies the smooth motion of instructions 8 and 9.

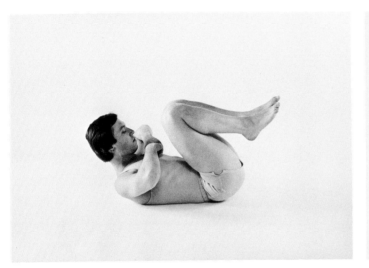 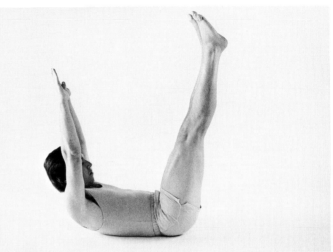

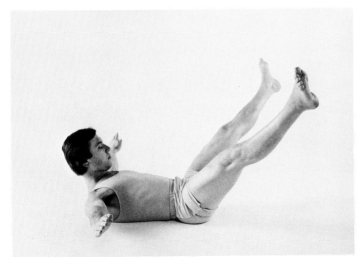 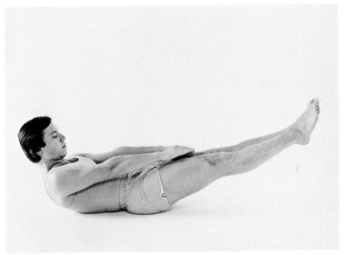

THIGH STRETCH I

Don't do this one if you have a knee problem.

Anchoring and Position

1. Kneel on the mat with your toes pointed, the tops of your feet on the mat.
2. Chin on chest.
3. Reach back carefully, one hand at a time, and take hold of your heels. Feel your chest lifted toward the ceiling, but don't arch your back.
4. Navel to spine. Very firm center. Pinch your bottom. Your body should be a single straight line from knees to shoulders.
5. You are anchored from your knees to your toes.

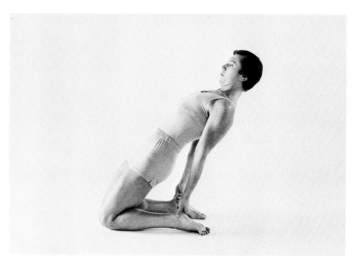

Movement

6. Lean backward, using your hands and arms to help control your motion. Keep your center firm and your body absolutely straight.
7. Lean only as far back as you can with complete control.
8. Reverse the motion, keeping your body straight and your chin on your chest. Return to Position.

Do up to three Thigh Stretches.

Breathing

Breathe IN on the way down.

OUT on the way up.

Checkpoints

1. Body absolutely straight. Navel to spine.
2. Chin on chest. Focus on your firm center.
3. Stay in control. Don't lean back too far.
4. You are a piece of iron. Do not bend or let your hips sink.

When you're good at the Thigh Stretch, consider moving on to this.

Anchoring and Position

1. Kneel on the mat with your toes pointed, the tops of your feet on the mat.
2. Chin on chest.
3. Navel to spine. Very firm center. Pinch your bottom. Your body should be a single straight line from knees to shoulders.
4. You are anchored from your knees to your toes.
5. Arms straight out in front of you, parallel to each other and to the mat. Reach long out of your shoulders with your fingers.

Movement

6. Keeping your center firm and body absolutely straight, lean slowly backward under full control. Keep reaching out of your shoulders with your fingers, and try to keep your arms more or less parallel to the mat.
7. Lean only as far back as you can with complete control.
8. Reverse the motion, keeping your body straight and your chin on your chest. Return to Position.

Do up to three Thigh Stretches.

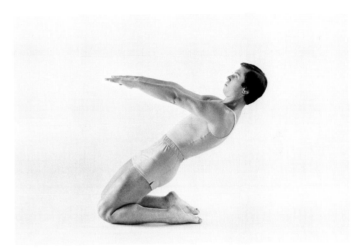

Breathing

Breathe IN on the way down.

OUT on the way up.

Checkpoints

1. Body absolutely straight. Navel to spine.
2. Chin on chest. Focus on your firm center.
3. Stay in control. Don't lean back too far.
4. You are a piece of iron. Do not bend or let your hips sink.
5. Reach with those fingers. They are a counterweight to your backward motion.

KNEE STRETCH

Position

1. Lie on your stomach, palms on the mat under your shoulders, legs straight, toes on the mat.
2. Navel to spine; firm center.
3. Push up, straightening your arms. Your body is one straight line.
4. Lift your left foot an inch or two off the mat, pointing your toe and stretching out of your hip. Lift your head and chest.

Movement

5. Bring your left knee to your chest. At the same time, curl your head down and in toward your center. Your navel is pressed to your spine; your back will round slightly.

6. Return to Position, stretching your leg out behind you and lifting your head and chest.

Do up to three Knee Stretches with your left leg and then do the same number with your right.

Breathing

Breathe IN as you stretch long.

OUT as you bring your head and knee in toward your center.

Checkpoints

1. Navel to spine.
2. Stationary leg straight.

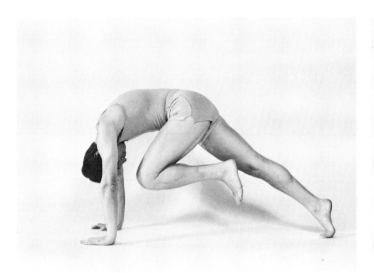 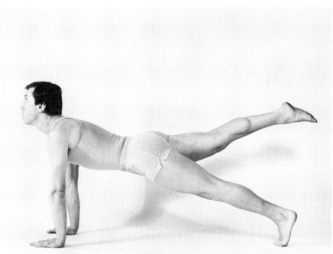

UPRIGHT CHAIR STRETCH

You will need an ordinary chair or stool, one with a wooden seat, if possible.

Position

1. Stand two feet or more from the chair. Put the ball of one foot flat on the edge of the chair seat. Adjust your position so that both legs are straight, your lifted toe softly pointed.

2. Navel to spine. Slide your head up the pole that runs up the center of your spine.

3. Lift your arms at your sides to shoulder height. Curve your arms and hands gracefully and bring them slightly forward, as if you were holding the world's largest, lightest beachball.

4. Feel a lightness and lift in your upper body, but don't arch your back or throw your chest out of line.

Movement

5. Keeping your back leg straight and your hips square, bend the knee of your raised leg. Your body should stay upright as it moves forward toward the chair. Arms shoulder height, still holding the beachball.

6. When you have gone as far forward as you can, stop. Feel the stretch in your straight leg. Your upper body is still light and lifted, your center firm.

7. Reverse the motion to return to Position.

Do three forward stretches.

Breathing

Breathe IN on the way forward.

OUT on the way back.

Checkpoints

1. Back leg straight.
2. Hips square. Back hip pressing forward.
3. Firm center. Body lifted.
4. Arms gracefully curved at shoulder height.
5. Don't hunch your shoulders.

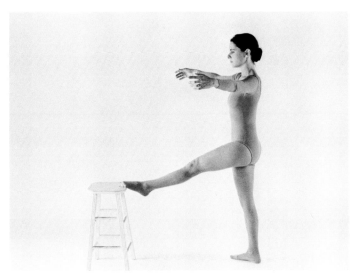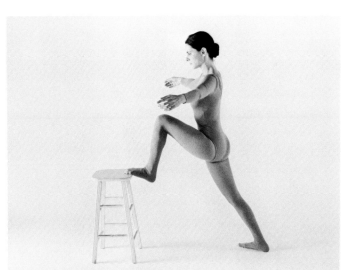

FORWARD CHAIR STRETCH

Another exercise you'll need a chair for. Or something like a chair.

Position

1. Stand about a foot and a half or two feet from the chair. Put the ball of your right foot flat on the edge of the chair or stool. Adjust your position so that your thigh is approximately level, your shin vertical.

2. Navel to spine. Slide your head up the imaginary pole that runs up the center of your spine.

3. Back leg straight, hip forward. Press into your heel.

4. Reaching out of your hips, lean forward and grasp the bottom of your foot with both hands. Arms straight.

Movement

5. In a single, smooth movement, straighten your bent leg and move your hips back, keeping them square. Keep your navel pressed to your spine, and let your back and head follow the movement naturally, pulling your head down close to your leg.

6. Stop when you are stretched to your limit, even if your bent leg isn't quite straight. The object is to have both legs straight and your head touching your leg, but don't strain. You will loosen into it gradually.

7. Reverse the motion to return to Position. Keep your back leg straight and your hips square.

Do three stretches on one leg, then change legs and do three more.

Breathing

Breathe IN as you stretch.

OUT as you return to Position.

Checkpoints

1. Back leg straight. Press into your heel.

2. Hips square. (Concentrate on pressing forward with the hipbone of your back leg.)

3. Firm center.

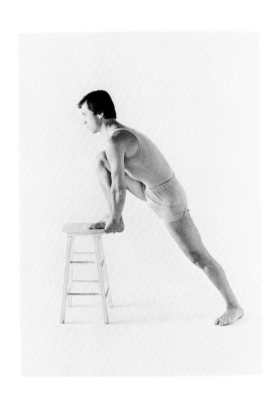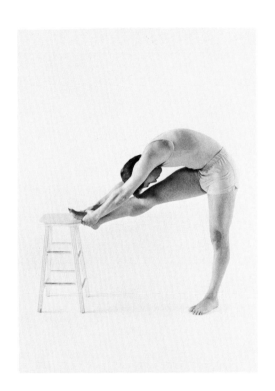

This one is a little complicated. It will help to do a dry run of the arm movements.

Position

1. Sit with your legs together and your hands at your sides. Feet flexed.
2. Navel to spine. Sit up out of your hips.
3. Feel yourself anchored to the mat from your heels to the base of your spine.
4. Begin to roll back, still sitting out of your hips. At the same time bring your chin to your chest, your elbows up and out and your knuckles to a point just under your chin.
5. Stop rolling back when your shoulders are about a foot off the mat. Keep your navel glued to your spine.

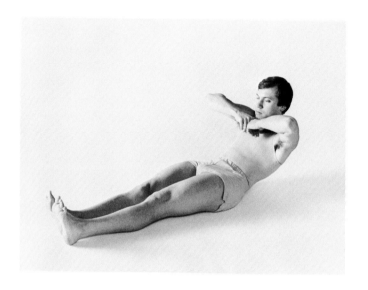

Movement

6. Holding your head and body motionless, extend your hands out at your sides so your arms are straight, in a line with each other and your shoulders.
7. Roll back up, at the same time bringing your straight arms around behind you (rotate your wrists). Clasp your hands if you can (do not interlace fingers) and keep pressing them upward. This will bring the top of your body forward.
8. When your (clasped) hands can go no higher, release them and keep rotating your straight arms up and around, in the largest circle your shoulder joint will allow. At the same time, keep curling your head in toward your center. Remember: navel to spine.
9. When your arms come around, reach out long toward and past your feet.
10. Uncurl into a sitting position and then, in the same

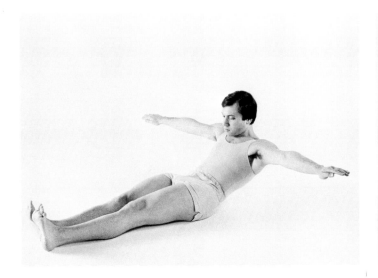
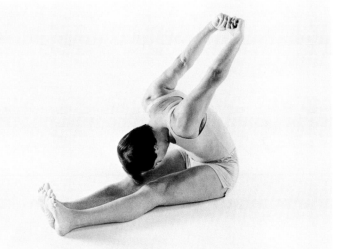

smooth movement, begin to roll down again, bringing your elbows out and hands up under your chin. Stop when you are in Position.

Do three Rowing movements.

Breathing

> Breathe IN as you roll backward.
>
> OUT as you curl forward.

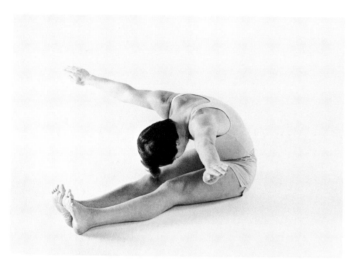
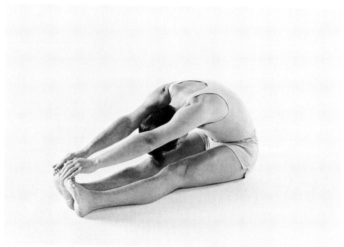

Checkpoints

1. Navel to spine. Firm center at all times.
2. Legs straight and together. Feet flexed.
3. Chin on chest.
4. Elbows up.
5. Really stretch and reach with your arms. Make the biggest circle you can.

THE BEANBAG

There is one piece of Pilates apparatus you can easily make for yourself. It's called the beanbag, because that's what it is. The basic exercise you do with it is good for strengthening your hands and toning your arms; done properly, it has all the other benefits of the method—firming your center, improving your posture, etc.

To make a beanbag, you'll need a bag. A cloth bag is best, but a sturdy plastic bag will do. You are going to fill it with three pounds of dried beans; it will not take a very big bag. The Pilates beanbag is about eight inches square when it's empty.

When the beans are in the bag, tie its neck securely with one end of a six-foot length of clothesline or similar cord, so that you can dangle the bag at the end of the cord and lift it up and down without worrying that it will drop off or spill.

For the other end of the cord, you'll need a piece of dowel between twelve and eighteen inches long, about an inch in diameter. A section of broomstick is a little too thin, but it's acceptable if there's no place where you can conveniently buy a piece of dowel. (Any store that stocks lumber should be able to help you, as should a well-stocked hardware store.)

The idea is to fasten the free end of the cord to the dowel so that when you turn the dowel, the rope winds around it

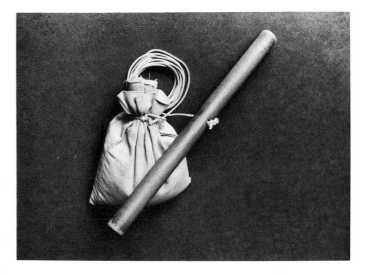

like thread on a spool. The best way to do this is by drilling a hole through the middle of the dowel, pushing the cord through the hole, and making a big knot in the end of the cord so it won't slip back through. If you don't have a drill and a vise, you can't do this. Next best would be to nail, screw, or staple the rope to the dowel.

That's all there is to it. Once you've done that, you have all the equipment you need to do the Beanbag.

You can do this standing on the mat, but it's better if you can stand on a telephone book or something else that will lift you a few inches off the floor.

Position

1. Wind all the cord around the middle of the rod. There should be room on either side of the cord for your hands.

2. Grasp the rod with both hands, one on each side of the rolled-up cord, so that the backs of your hands and your knuckles are on top of the rod when you extend your arms.

3. Hold your arms out in front of you so that your elbows are straight. Reach out of your shoulders but do not let them rise. The rod should be parallel to the floor at shoulder level.

4. Hold yourself tall by firming your center.

Movement

5. The idea is to unroll the cord so the beanbag makes its way toward the floor. Do this by moving one hand at a time:

    (a) Curl your left wrist and hand downward, letting the rod rotate in your right hand. This should re-lease some cord. If it doesn't, turn the rod around and start again.

    (b) Next, curl your right wrist down and let the rod rotate in your left hand. The beanbag should progress farther toward the floor. Keep your arms straight and level.

    (c) Alternate hands until the beanbag reaches the floor, if you can.

6. Now reverse to bring the beanbag back up. This time:

    (a) Open one hand and curl it downward, holding the rod with the other so that it doesn't rotate.

    (b) Close your hand and flex the curled wrist backward to rotate the rod so the cord winds around it.

    (c) Alternate hands until the beanbag is all the way up to the rod.

Do this once only. After you've been doing it once for a long time, try doing it twice. If you can do it three times, congratulations! (At first, you may not be able to do it once. In that case, only let the beanbag halfway to the floor before winding it back up. As you get better at it, gradually increase the amount as you lower it.)

Breathing

Breathe IN and OUT naturally, in rhythm with the way your hands are moving.

Checkpoints

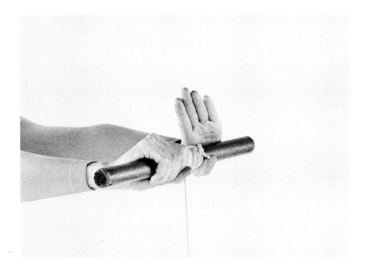

1. Get the maximum rotation in your wrist each time you curl or flex it.
2. Arms straight.
3. Stand up tall. Slide your head up that pole.
4. Arms level; shoulders level.
5. Don't hunch your shoulders.
6. Firm center.

A fabulous relaxer. Do standing up or sitting down.

Position

1. (a) If you are standing: navel to spine. Firm center.

   (b) If you are sitting: sit up tall out of your hips.

2. Shrug your shoulders high toward your ears.

3. Release those muscles so your shoulders drop.

4. Think of those muscles getting still looser. Let your shoulders fall farther.

Movement

5. Think of your neck as being a long, elastic stalk. Bring your head forward. Feel the stretch in your neck. Your head is very heavy—it is making your neck longer. Let your head hang, pulling on your neck, for a few moments.

6. Lift your head slowly and, with control, let it drop to one side the way it dropped forward, getting heavier as it pulls toward your shoulder.

7. Lift your head again and do the same thing to the other side.

8. Now let it move backward. Do this very slowly and gradually, maintaining control and letting your neck stretch only a little at a time, until you can relax it without hurting yourself.

9. Lift your head again. Repeat instruction number 5. This time roll your head to the left, letting its weight stretch your neck the whole way. Make the biggest circle you can with the top of your head.

10. Reverse and roll it once in the other direction.

Breathing

(a) Lift and stretch:

Breathe IN as you lift your head.

OUT as you stretch your neck.

(b) Rolling:

Breathe IN for the first half of the circle.

Force all the air from your lungs as you complete the circle with your head.

BEND AND STRETCH

Position

1. Stand with your feet shoulder-width apart.
2. Clasp your hands behind your back.
3. Navel to spine. Firm center, lifted chest. Stand tall.

Movement

4. Constantly pulling your navel to your spine, lift your arms behind you. Keep them straight.
5. As your arms rise, let your head drop forward and down. Chin on chest. Begin to bend at the waist.
6. Concentrate on lifting your arms toward the ceiling and beyond while pulling your navel to your spine. Keep your legs straight. This will force you to bend more and more, bringing your head closer to your legs. Feel the stretch through your neck, back and legs.
7. Stop when you can go no farther, or when you feel strain.
8. Reverse the motion slowly and with control to return to Position.

Bend and Stretch three times.

Breathing

Breathe IN on the way up.

   OUT as you bend forward.

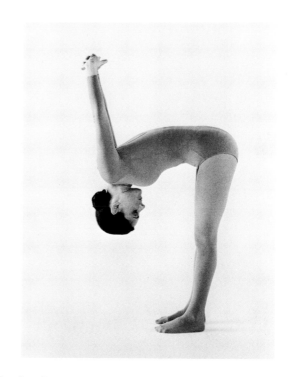

Checkpoints

1. Navel to spine.
2. Legs straight.
3. The motive power is in your arms.
4. Keep the motion smooth in both directions. Don't jerk down.

This can be hard on your knees. Be careful.

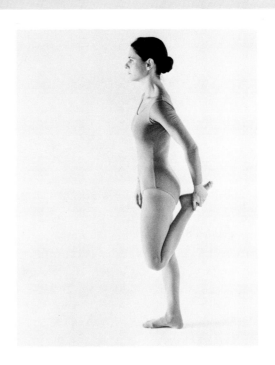

Position and Movement

1. Stand with your feet shoulder-width apart.
2. Bend your left knee to bring your heel back and close to your buttocks. At the same time reach down and grasp your instep.
3. Straighten up again. Shoulders and hips level. Right leg straight.
4. Navel to spine. Firm center. Lift your chest and slide your head up the pole that runs through your spine.
5. Pull your foot toward your buttocks. Try to make the heel touch.
6. Relax.

Do three Thigh Stretches. Change legs and do three more.

Breathing

Breathe IN as you pull.

OUT as you relax.

Checkpoints

1. Tall and thin. Firm center.
2. Hips and shoulders level.
3. Still as a statue when you pull and relax.

OFFICE-WALL PLIÉ

Pick an empty wall or a door in your office. You'll need enough room to extend both arms along the wall. Be careful not to swat any pictures, furniture, or co-workers.

Position

1. Stand with your heels together, against the wall, your toes spread.
2. Arms straight out at your sides, against the wall. Reach out of your shoulders, but don't let them rise.
3. Navel to spine. Spine to wall.
4. Stretch your neck long and press the base of your skull to the wall.

Movement

5. Bend your knees and slide your back down the wall as far as you can. Go up on your toes, but keep your heels pressed against the wall.

6. Smoothly reverse the motion and return to Position.

Plié three to five times.

Breathing

Breathe IN on the way down.

OUT on the way up.

Checkpoints

1. Heels together and against wall.
2. Neck long.
3. Spine flat against the wall. Firm center.
4. Don't hunch your shoulders.

REACH FOR THE SKY

As long as you're standing by that clear stretch of wall, here's another.

Position

1. Stand with your back against the wall, your heels out from the wall about a foot, your legs straight.
2. Arms straight out at your sides. Reach out of your shoulders but don't let them rise.
3. Navel to spine. Spine to wall.
4. Neck long. Press the base of your skull against the wall.

Movement

5. Smoothly raise your arms overhead, keeping them against the wall the whole way if you can, reaching out of your shoulders. Don't let your back arch away from the wall.

6. Reverse the motion to return to Position.

Reach three to five times.

Breathing

Breathe IN as you reach upward.

Press the air from your lungs as you bring your arms down.

Checkpoints

1. Back flat against the wall at all times. FLAT!
2. Don't hunch your shoulders.

THE ROLL-DOWN

A vertical version of the Roll-Up that lets you keep your clothes clean.

Position

1. Stand with your back pressed flat against the wall. Heels six to eight inches from the wall. Arms at your sides.
2. Navel to spine, spine to wall.

Movement

3. Pressing your navel to your spine at all times, roll your head forward. Stretch your neck long.
4. When your chin is on your chest, let your shoulders come away from the wall. Your arms are relaxed, your fingers reaching very gently for the floor.
5. Roll your back away from the wall one vertebra at a time. When your head is pointing at the floor, relax your neck.
6. Roll down as far as you can. Keep your bottom against the wall.

7. Roll up to Position, using the muscles of your center to press first one vertebra and then the next against the wall.

Roll down and up again three to five times.

NOTE: Don't confuse this exercise with toe-touching. Done properly, especially in combination with a Head Roll and Reach for the Sky, it can really wake you up.

Breathing

Breathe IN on the way UP.

> OUT on the way down. Force the last drop of air from your lungs before you start up.

Checkpoints

1. Navel to spine! It's the magic ingredient.
2. Chin on chest only at the beginning. Go with gravity.
3. As you get better, start with your heels closer to the wall.

You don't need as much wall (or door) for this one, which is especially valuable for skiers.

Position

1. Stand with your back against the wall, your feet a little more than a foot from the wall, your legs straight.
2. Navel to spine. Spine to wall.
3. Neck long; press the base of your skull to the wall.

Movement

4. Bend your legs and let your back slide down the wall until your thighs are level, as if you were sitting in a chair. Your hands can be at your sides or on your thighs.
5. Hold that way as long as you can. You'll feel it in your thighs.
6. Straighten your legs and slide back up into Position.

One is enough. Do up to three if you want to.

Variations

1. When you get good at this, try lifting one foot straight out ahead of you when you get down into the Imaginary Chair. Alternate.
2. *Before* you start to slide down, extend one foot straight in front of you. Then slide down, hold, and slide back up. Put your foot down. Alternate.

Breathing

Breathe IN on the way down.

OUT and IN (and OUT and IN) naturally while you hold in the chair.

OUT on the way up.

Checkpoints

1. Back absolutely flat against the wall.
2. Navel to spine. Firm center.
3. Don't overdo it.

Something to do while walking up to the top of the Empire State Building, on the front steps of your house, or the hall stairs outside your office. (Or use a book or two.)

Position

1. Put one foot a step higher than the other. Upper foot: ball of the toe on the edge of the stair tread, heel up as high as it will go. Lower foot: flat on the stair tread.
2. Put your hands on top of your head, elbows out to the side. (Or, one hand on your head, hold the banister with the other.)

Movement

3. Rise up on the toe of your lower foot, feeling the lift right along your spine and neck, as if you were being pulled up by a rope attached to the top of your head. Keep your chest high.
4. Return to Position smoothly and with control, lifting as you lower.

Do three lifts on one foot, then three on the other. (Go up a step each time, if you want.)

Variations

Do the same movement

1. with your upper foot flat on the stair tread
2. with the ball of your upper foot on the stair tread and your heel pushed down as low as you can get it

Breathing

Breathe IN as you lift.

OUT as you return to Position.

Checkpoints

1. Firm center. Body straight and tall.
2. Keep your balance.
3. Lift at all times.

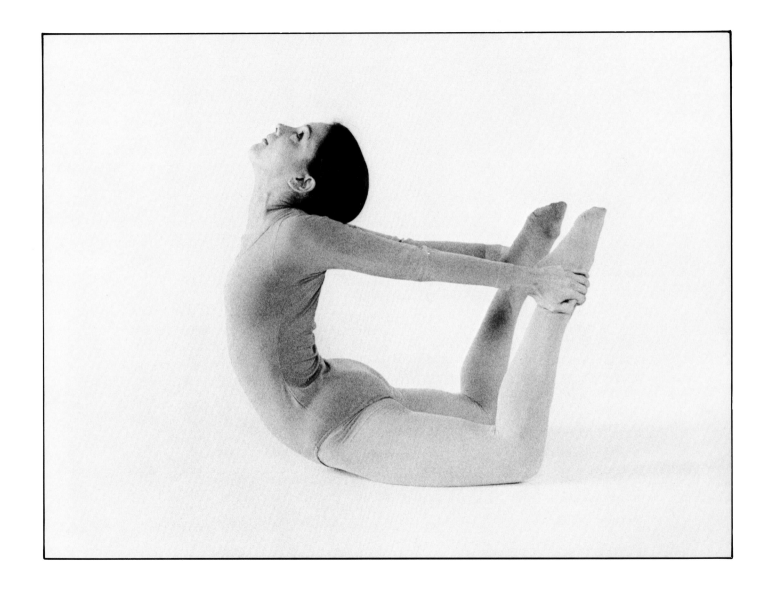

CHAPTER TEN

New Body, New Life

The Pilates Method will change your body, and it will change your life. It is not a fad or the subject of a new and fleeting cult. It is a system that has proved its value over the years, drawing and holding among its adherents people whose need for suppleness, muscle tone, grace, and harmony of mind and body goes considerably beyond that of the average gymgoer.

New Bodies, and Reconditioned Ones, Too

An indication of how well the Pilates Method can work in giving you a new body is its use in rehabilitation.

Prominent among the physicians who are familiar with the Pilates Method's therapeutic value are Dr. William Hamilton and Dr. Willibald Nagler. Dr. Hamilton is the official orthopedic surgeon of the New York City Ballet and the School of American Ballet. He repairs injuries sustained by their dancers, as well as members of the Joffrey Ballet, the American Ballet Theater, and other companies from all over the country. Dr. Nagler is head of rehabilitative medicine (Physiatrist-in-Chief) at the New York Hospital–Cornell Medical Center. He, too, works with dancers and with athletes.

For both Dr. Hamilton and Dr. Nagler, the Pilates Method has proved its value in the restoration of strength and endurance, two of the prime goals of rehabilitative medicine.

When he suggests the Pilates Method to his patients, Dr. Hamilton makes no extravagant claims, preferring to let the patients see for themselves if the method works for them. The response, he reports, is remarkably uniform. Typical is the patient who called to say, "The best thing you ever did for me was to send me to Pilates, and I'm going back there for the rest of my life."

Dr. Hamilton finds the method valuable not only for rehabilitation after surgery, but as a way to avoid surgery entirely. For example, he says, it can be used to provide strengthening and the control necessary for accurate placement of the leg, so that a patient (a dancer, for instance) can protect a minor tear in a knee cartilage well enough to make surgery unnecessary.

Besides repairing injuries and restoring lost function, Dr. Hamilton and Dr. Nagler are intent on preventing reinjury. Identifying and removing the cause of the injury is vital, but in the past, Dr. Nagler points out, paying attention only to the sick part of the body sometimes resulted in general deconditioning. Now it is accepted that an important element in preventing reinjury is proper conditioning not just of the injured area but of the whole body. Imbalances and weak points in the body can be major sources of trouble. "If you push any musculoskeletal structure long enough and hard enough," says Dr. Hamilton, "you'll find its weak links."

Few of us tax our bodies as much as ballet dancers or professional athletes do, but we are all subject to physical stress, and we are all open to injury. If we are to avoid it, we—like dancers and athletes—have to be properly conditioned.

A simple but significant example was provided by Dr. Nagler: balance in posture—one of the Pilates Method's primary goals and results—eliminates a lot of aches and pains. Especially backaches.

Our sessions at the Pilates Studio are frequently shared with people (of all ages and professions) who have come to correct problems they have with their knees or feet, with their hips, with their hands or arms, and—most commonly—with their backs. Among them is actress Candice Bergen. "The Pilates Method is the first thing that has worked for my back," she says. "It has strengthened the areas that needed to be helped. As long as I keep doing the work, I don't have to go to back doctors at all."

While we are confident that the Pilates Method can prevent and relieve the kind of muscular discomfort that seems epidemic these days, we do not recommend that you use this book to prescribe a course of rehabilitative therapy for yourself. If you already have aches and pains (back pains, in particular), you should be especially careful. Consult your doctor about the exercises in this book. With his help, you can come up with a program you will be able to follow safely.

Even if you think of yourself as being reasonably fit when you start the Pilates Method, you will find as you progress that you are becoming aware of weaknesses and imbalances you never knew you had. Focus on them. Do your best to maintain balance in all the movements. (If, for instance, you tend to lean to one side, try to counteract it.) With time, the weakness or imbalance will diminish and disappear.

Pilates and Sports

Pilates regulars are unanimous in reporting that the method has helped their sports performance. Tennis and squash are sports frequently mentioned, as are running, skiing, and skating. Everyone notes an improvement in control, coordination, and endurance. Some people find that their reaction time improves.

The value of the method's general balancing and conditioning effect is easiest to see in sports which call for a symmetrical use of the body (running, skiing, skating, swimming, gymnastics, basketball). But in a sense it is even more important for sports which emphasize one side of the body over another (tennis and other racket sports, for example). Their stress on skills training neglects over-all fitness, which is vital to coordination and agility and which protects against injuries due to abrupt movement.

The human body is ill-suited to sudden physical stress, especially when it is unprepared. We've heard since childhood about the importance of warming up before engaging in any strenuous activity. Warming up, of course, hasn't got much to do with temperature. It's a matter of gradually getting the muscles into action, loosening and stretching them, building your pulse rate, beginning to breathe deeper. Preparing the body for the demands that are going to be put on it.

There is no better warmup than a short session of Pilates exercises. (Ballet, beyond its artistic component, is one of the most intense and competitive forms of athletics, and the Pilates Method is regularly used as warmup for ballet. Suzanne Farrell told us, "I usually do some of the exercises after I get to the theater early in the day, and then I do some before the performance.")

While almost everyone has heard how important it is to warm up, cooling off properly after strenuous activity has had much less attention. It can be dangerous simply to stop after a hard game of tennis or miles of running. Stopping too abruptly can have a variety of bad effects, some of them serious. If you're lucky, you'll get away with only stiffness and pain.

When you're ready to quit, instead of heading straight for the shower (or, worse yet, just sitting down), spend ten minutes or more with the Pilates Method. You'll be amazed at the difference it makes in how you feel afterward.

By and large, you shouldn't isolate the movements from the method, but we do have a few suggestions for exercises that are especially useful for specific sports.

Joggers and runners will benefit especially from exercises that stretch their legs. For cooling off, in particular, the Forward Chair Stretch is a good way to keep from stiffening up. Outdoors, it can be done with the raised foot against a tree or fence post or parking meter, or propped atop a fireplug. Remember to keep your back leg straight as you bend forward. The Push-Up gives a good stretch to the backs of your legs if you pay special attention to keeping your heels on the ground. You don't even have to do the pushing up part of the exercise; just walk in and out on your hands. The stairway exercises are also good. Do them whenever you're on a stairway; use a curb or the roots of a tree just before and after you run.

All of these exercises will be similarly helpful for skiers and skaters. Skiers should also take note of the Imaginary Chair: it is a potent thigh strengthener.

For tennis and other racket sports, we recommend the Beanbag. There is some evidence that strong wrists and forearms may help prevent tennis elbow; in any case, they certainly help your stroke.

Golfers will find that the Saw and the Spine Twist help them get their shoulders and body around for backswing and follow through. And regular sessions of the Pilates Method will make a big difference in their ability to keep their eyes on the ball.

Using What You Know

It may be that you have some favorite exercises you want to keep doing in addition to the Pilates Method. If so, remember that you've been learning not just a specific group of exercises, but a whole new way of thinking about movement. You'll get a lot more out of whatever you do if you apply the Pilates principles to it.

Before you do an exercise, take a moment to analyze it. What are you really doing? Should you have your spine to the mat? Or sit up out of your hips? Certainly, whatever the movement, you don't want to let your stomach bulge or your shoulders hunch up. You want to concentrate, to maintain full control. To establish and maintain a firm center. To move smoothly and with precision, and to coordinate your breathing with the movement. (Breathing in at the point of effort or when the movement naturally compresses your lungs.)

The Method in Bed

It has become a commonplace observation that people who are fit have a better sex life than people who aren't. There are several reasons for this, the simplest being that sex requires a certain amount of sustained physical exertion. Also, if your body is in good physical shape, it looks good and you feel better about it, so you're less likely to experience embarrassment or anxiety or other mental discomfort about sex. This is all well and good, as far as it goes. And, as far as it goes, it all applies to the Pilates Method.

But there is an important flaw in it. The correlation between fitness and sex, as it is seen by exercise-for-sex advocates, is essentially mechanistic—a matter of athletics. Like the exercises themselves, this emphasizes the physical without including the mental. You become an observer when, more than any other time, you should be a participant.

If you talk to psychiatrists and psychologists who do sex therapy (the reputable ones), you will learn that "spectatoring" in this way is one of the prime barriers to full sexual functioning and enjoyment. And here, the Pilates Method does something uniquely helpful. By training you to be intimately aware of your body, to merge your mental and physical processes instead of separating them, it facilitates a non-observational body sense that can be a great heightener of sexual pleasure. It is not only your appearance and your stamina that can be improved, but the depth and degree of your participation.

New Life

"In with the air, out with the air. Sit tall, taller. Out of your hips. Long the legs. Pinch, pinch, pinch."

Instructions you'll only hear at the Pilates Studio, so ingrained by Joe that his old-country phrases come out of the mouths of second-generation instructors who know him only as a legend.

We cannot bring the studio to you, but we have tried to impart its essence.

You have in your hands a kind of basic tool. If you put your mind to it, it can mold and shape your body, firm muscles you never knew you had, take off unwanted inches. It can make you graceful. It can help you look and feel younger. You can develop a new balance, not just physical but mental.

Some changes will be noticeable almost immediately; others will take longer, but they will happen.

The world will seem a different place, and you a different person in it.